The Pregnancy Test

150 Important, Embarrassing, and Slightly Neurotic Questions

by Melissa Heckscher
with Emily Sikking, M.D.

QUIRK BOOKS
PHILADELPHIA

Disclaimer: The authors made every effort to present accurate information about pregnancy and childbirth, but a book is never a substitute for a living, breathing physician. Always consult your doctor if you have questions or concerns about your pregnancy.

Copyright © 2011 Melissa Hecksher

Library of Congress Cataloging in Publication Number: 2010936313

ISBN: 978-1-59474-475-4

Printed in China

Typeset in Century Schoolbook

Designed by Jenny Kraemer
Production management by John J. McGurk

Published by Quirk Books
215 Church Street
Philadelphia, PA 19106
www.quirkbooks.com

10 9 8 7 6 5 4 3 2 1

Introduction

Pregnancy is an exciting time. But it is also a scary time, filled with suddenly urgent questions: Can you go to the gym? *(Sure.)* Can you have a glass of wine? *(On special occasions, maybe.)* Can you eat a spicy tuna roll or a spoonful of raw cookie dough? *(Not good ideas.)* Basically, can you lead the life you used to without endangering the health of your growing baby? *(Yes, but with a few minor adjustments.)* It's a big responsibility, and *The Pregnancy Test* is here to help.

We are first-hand experts on the subject. One of us (Melissa) was a paranoid pregnant woman (who's now a paranoid mother). The other (Emily) is a trusted ob-gyn. In this handy volume we strive to answer some of the most important, embarrassing, obscure, and occasionally neurotic questions about pregnancy and childbirth that women have ever asked.

Part trivia game, part prescription, *The Pregnancy Test* is a combination of medical facts and doctor-dispensed advice. The questions came from the authors, their pregnant friends or patients, and online pregnancy forums. The answers were compiled using a variety of sources, including the American College of Obstetricians and Gynecologists, the March of Dimes, and a litany of published research articles (as well as Emily's own expert brain).

So if you've ever wondered whether your nether regions will survive childbirth unscathed, turn to page 241. Or if you want to know whether your growing belly will inhibit your having sex, see page 237. Or if you should avoid riding roller coasters or leave jumping out of an airplane to another day (pages 9 and 179)—you'll find these questions and their answers (and many more) within.

But this test is meant for your education and entertainment. No one's keeping score. You can play the book like a game or read it like a novel. Quiz your Lamaze buddies or enlighten your spouse. There are no rules here.

Most important: Have fun. Not just while reading this book, but always. Enjoy your pregnancy. Enjoy your baby. Yes, being pregnant is stressful. Yes, having a baby is a big responsibility. Yes, you've got to watch what you eat-drink-and-do for nine months. But don't let your deluge of questions obstruct the big picture. Being a happy parent makes a happy child.

Remember that this is just the beginning. You've got a long, crazy, wonderful journey ahead of you. Congratulations!

1

What could happen if I drink alcohol before knowing I'm pregnant?

❏ a.   You may stunt the baby's growth.
❏ b.   Probably nothing, but lay off the booze.
❏ c.   You will cause birth defects.
❏ d.   It won't hurt the baby, but since your body
         can't process alcohol when you're pregnant,
         even a little alcohol might damage your liver.

Answer:

b.

According to the March of Dimes, a baby's brain and other organs begin developing about the fifth week of pregnancy (a week after your missed period and around a week after a home pregnancy test would show a positive result). As long as you put down that mojito before this crucial period, everything will likely be fine. Even if you consume some alcohol after this time, the odds are in your favor that your baby would be OK.

But now that you know you're pregnant, it's best to practice teetotalism. Although an occasional sip of wine probably won't adversely affect your baby, some studies have linked even a moderate amount of alcohol use to miscarriages. Heavy drinking may lead to fetal alcohol syndrome, a condition that can cause flattened facial features and lifelong learning disabilities.

The more you drink, the greater the risk. Experts say risks to the fetus are highest with binge drinking (consuming so much liquor that you black out) and for those women who consume seven or more drinks per week.

#2

What if I get pregnant while I'm on the birth control pill?

❏ a.   The added hormones could affect the baby's sexual development.

❏ b.   It's not the hormones you have to worry about, it's the added chemicals.

❏ c.   It likely won't affect the baby at all, as long as you stop taking the pill now.

❏ d.   The added estrogen in the pill could make your baby more emotional.

Answer:

C.

Experts estimate that 1 to 5 percent of women accidentally use oral contraceptives during the first part of their pregnancies, thereby exposing their unborn children to the artificial estrogens that are intended to prevent conception.

But according to the American College of Obstetricians and Gynecologists, taking birth control pills during pregnancy doesn't increase the risk of birth defects. In the past, concerns were raised that some oral contraceptives (those containing higher doses of hormones, in particular) could interfere with the development of a baby's sex organs, but today's lower-dose pills pose no such risk.

Still, you should stop birth control medication once you learn you're pregnant. A 2009 University of Ottawa study found that women who continued past the first trimester were more likely to deliver preterm or have babies with low birth weights. If you stopped taking the pill as soon as you found out you were pregnant, your baby is most likely fine. But if you're concerned, ask your doctor to monitor your baby's development to ensure everything is normal and healthy.

#3

Can I ride
a roller coaster?

❑ a.   Sure, as long as you don't go upside down.
❑ b.   No, sharp turns can cause the baby's
        umbilical cord to tangle, interrupting blood
        and oxygen flow to your baby.
❑ c.   No, the roller coaster's sudden starts and
        stops can rip the placenta from the uterine
        wall, which can be dangerous for you and
        your baby.
❑ d.   No, sudden ups and downs can jostle your
        baby and affect brain development.

Answer:

C.

The shearing forces exerted on a woman's womb by roller coasters are the same as those present in car crashes. Such rapid starts and stops can cause the placenta to rip away from the wall of the uterus, which cuts off the flow of oxygen and nutrients to the baby. This condition, called placental abruption, is an emergency for both mother and baby.

Placental abruption is less likely to happen in the first 12 weeks of pregnancy, because the placenta is not fully developed and is therefore less likely to be jarred out of place. So if you can't abstain entirely from amusement park rides, indulging in them earlier in your pregnancy is better. Still, your best bet is to stick to the kiddie rides—the carousel, swings, and Ferris wheel are safe for your pregnant body—until after your baby is born. Then you'll have a whole different kind of roller coaster to ride.

What causes morning sickness?

❏ a.   Nausea and vomiting is your body's way of trying to reject the baby.

❏ b.   Since your baby is taking so many of your nutrients, your body is left malnourished, which causes nausea.

❏ c.   Many women tend to change their diets dramatically during pregnancy, which causes an upset stomach.

❏ d.   Nobody knows for sure, though it likely has to do with hormones.

Answer:

d.

Scientists aren't completely sure what causes morning sickness, though many believe it is triggered by the rapid rise in the level of hormones needed to help the growth of the placenta and fetus during early pregnancy. Here's what we do know:

- It occurs only in humans.
- It doesn't only happen in the morning.
- It's often triggered by the smell and taste of foods historically likely to cause food-borne illnesses, as well as by cigarette smoke and alcohol.
- It usually peaks between 6 and 18 weeks of pregnancy—a period during which the fetus is particularly vulnerable to toxic chemicals.

For these reasons, some scientists think morning sickness is an adaptive function designed to prevent a pregnant woman from eating or drinking something that could adversely affect her unborn baby. Vomiting at the first whiff of hard liquor, for instance, is a pretty good deterrent to downing a few shots after dinner.

About two-thirds of mommies-to-be experience morning sickness. If you're among the one-third who don't, consider yourself lucky.

I'm not experiencing morning sickness. What does that mean?

❏ a.   You're more likely to be carrying a boy.
❏ b.   Your body may be less sensitive to pregnancy's hormonal changes.
❏ c.   You are more likely to miscarry or have other pregnancy complications.
❏ d.   You're probably not eating enough.

Answer:
b.

Doctors have long said that morning sickness is a sign of a healthy pregnancy, but being nausea-free doesn't mean that your pregnancy will have problems. In fact, more than a third of all pregnant women don't experience morning sickness (which doesn't always happen in the morning, by the way; see question #4), and studies have shown that they are no more likely to miscarry than others.

So why do some pregnant women spend their first trimester nauseated while others remain puke-free? Probably because we're all different. The nausea is thought to be caused by a rise in estrogen levels during early pregnancy. Since every woman's prepregnancy hormone levels vary, sudden increases may affect some women more than others.

Basically, if you're not spending the first few weeks taming your gag reflex, be thankful!

Can my throwing up strain my baby?

❏ a. The act of vomiting doesn't, but excessive vomiting can cause other problems.

❏ b. In severe cases, the stomach muscles can clench and deprive the baby of oxygen.

❏ c. Extremely forceful heaves can trigger labor, even if you're weeks from your due date.

❏ d. Your baby's brain development can be affected since the act of vomiting shakes the entire body, including the uterus.

Answer:

a.

Rest assured that your baby is well protected within the muscular walls of the uterus, no matter how violently ill you may feel. As in a grueling abdominal workout, your stomach muscles contract when you vomit, which is why you may feel sore afterward. Make sure you're staying hydrated, drinking enough water to compensate for all the fluids you're losing. Dehydration can be bad for your baby (and you).

If you're so nauseous that you can't keep any food or liquids down, call your doctor. This condition, experienced by 1 to 2 percent of pregnant women, is called hyperemesis gravidarum and can be dangerous for both mother and baby. Severe cases require hospitalization so that the mother can get fluid and nutrients through an intravenous line.

Contact your doctor if you experience

- vomiting that is accompanied by pain or fever
- nausea/vomiting that extends into the second trimester
- signs of dehydration, including lightheadedness and dark-colored or infrequent urine
- weight loss

Don't worry, though, you should feel better soon. Morning sickness usually goes away by the 18th week of pregnancy.

True or False:

You can become pregnant while you're already pregnant.

Answer:

true.

This phenomenon, called superfetation, occurs when a woman ovulates twice in a given menstrual cycle. It differs from twin pregnancies, which are the result of two eggs being released at one time.

Superfetation is so rare that only 10 cases have ever been documented. Among them are British couple Amelia Spence and George Herrity, who in 2007 conceived two girls three weeks apart. According to newspaper reports, the first baby weighed 6 pounds, 11 ounces after 32 weeks in the womb; the second weighed 4 pounds, 13 ounces after 29 weeks in the womb. More recently, in 2009 Arkansas couple Todd and Julia Grovenburg conceived two babies—a boy and a girl—two and a half weeks apart.

True or False:

A baby who develops outside the uterus cannot survive.

Answer:
false.

It is possible for a fetus to develop outside the uterus, but it's unlikely to be a healthy baby. Ectopic pregnancies occur when a fertilized egg implants in the fallopian tubes or, less commonly, the ovaries. Usually, such pregnancies either miscarry because the embryo cannot properly grow or are terminated by doctors because of the fatal risk they pose to the mother.

But at least one baby has survived an ectopic pregnancy. In 2008, a 34-year-old Australian woman gave birth two weeks early to a healthy 6-pound, 3-ounce baby girl who had developed in the ovary. Doctors somehow missed the condition because the woman reportedly showed no symptoms of an ectopic pregnancy and the location of the fetus was unclear on an ultrasound.

Early on, it may be hard to distinguish an ectopic pregnancy from a normal one, but as the pregnancy progresses, it's hard to miss. Symptoms associated with the former include abdominal or pelvic pain, vaginal bleeding, painful intercourse, dizziness, fainting, and shoulder pain caused by bleeding under the diaphragm.

My doctor says my baby weighs only 1 pound, so why have I gained 15?

❑ a.　　Blood, breasts, and baby fat are heavy baggage.
❑ b.　　Pregnancy slows your metabolism.
❑ c.　　The placenta weighs 14 pounds.
❑ d.　　Too many Twinkies.

Answer:

a.

It's not just your baby that's getting bigger. Pregnancy packs on pounds in ways you probably never imagined (all of which are temporary, provided you don't overdo it with the late-night ice cream cravings). As early as the tenth week, hormonal fluctuations will likely add a pound or two onto your boobs alone. From then on, you'll probably gain about seven pounds of fat (reserves for your baby in case you skip a few meals) and eight pounds of added blood volume and retained fluids.

All told, your body will have accumulated about 30 pounds by the time you give birth. Here's the breakdown:

Baby: 7 to 8 pounds
Placenta: 1 to 2 pounds
Amniotic fluid: 2 pounds
Uterus: 2 pounds
Maternal breast tissue: 2 pounds
Maternal blood: 4 pounds
Fluids in maternal tissue: 4 pounds
Maternal fat and nutrient stores: 7 pounds

#10

What if I experience weird spasms in my belly? What does that mean?

- ❏ a.   Your baby may be having seizures.
- ❏ b.   Your baby may have gas.
- ❏ c.   Your baby may have the hiccups.
- ❏ d.   Your baby may be coughing.

Answer:

C.

Between 24 and 28 weeks, most pregnant women start to feel the rhythmic thumps of their babies' hiccups. There's no need to worry—hiccups are common both in and out of the womb. In fact, many doctors believe them to be a sign of healthy fetal nervous and respiratory systems.

Nobody knows for sure why these hiccuping episodes happen; however, doctors generally agree that most are triggered by breathing or swallowing amniotic fluid (which is normal). These watery intakes cause fluid to flow into and out of the lungs, which in turn causes the diaphragm to contract and hiccuping to ensue. Regular, extrauterine hiccups are caused by similar contractions of the diaphragm.

Another reason to love those little thumps in your belly: A 2007 University of Kansas study suggested that hiccups may regulate the fetal heart during the third trimester. So while those rhythmic spasms in your abdomen might be a bit uncomfortable, they're a good thing for your little one.

On the other hand, there's no evidence showing that a lack of fetal hiccups is a sign of problems. Hiccuping episodes can happen several times a day—or not at all.

#11

As my baby grows, what's happening to my organs?

❑ a.   They shrink to make room for your baby.
❑ b.   They move to make room for your baby.
❑ c.   Your small intestine is no longer needed during pregnancy.
❑ d.   Only your bladder gets smaller. The rest of your organs stay as is.

Answer:

b.

Simply put: Your organs make way for baby. Though it may seem like there's not enough space to accommodate an entire human being in addition to all your other parts, the female body is designed to do so. The organs that once occupied the area below your rib cage will shift and move to make room.

The intestinal tract does the bulk of the changing, since it took up most of the space in there before you conceived. As your baby gets bigger, your stomach will be pushed up toward your ribs and your bladder will be pushed down toward your rectum. Both organs will also (temporarily) get smaller, which explains both your frequent heartburn and frequent bathroom breaks.

#12

Why do I sometimes pee a little when I laugh?

❑ a.   Because pregnancy causes bladder infections.

❑ b.   Because pregnancy widens the walls of the urethra, so there's more room for urine to escape.

❑ c.   Because your baby is irritated by your laughter.

❑ d.   Because the uterus is sitting on your bladder, and everything pushes down when you laugh, sneeze, or cough.

Answer:

d.

When you laugh, your abdominal muscles tighten and your uterus, which is located directly on top of your bladder, pushes down just enough to send out a little bit of urine. Coughing, sneezing, or a particularly strong kick from your baby may have the same effect.

Unfortunately, there's not much you can do to prevent it from happening. Such leakage should stop once your baby is born, and daily Kegel exercises may hasten its departure. To do Kegels, simply tighten the same muscles you use to stop the flow of urine and hold five to ten seconds. Do several sets of ten a few times daily.

#13

Can my baby's kicking damage my internal organs?

❑ a. No, but if your baby is longer than 20 inches, a strong kick could puncture the amniotic sac and cause early labor.

❑ b. Yes. Kicking may puncture your lung.

❑ c. Possibly. If your baby is head-down, a strong kick could fracture one of your ribs.

❑ d. Kicks won't hurt you, but they could make you pee your pants.

Answer:

d.

Your uterus is strong enough to protect your baby from harm and your internal organs from even the most forceful of your baby's movements. Sure, it may feel like she's practicing kick-boxing techniques on your bladder; but the truth is, her kicks aren't strong enough to do any damage.

That's not to say they don't hurt. Strong kicks or punches may hit your bladder, cervix, or bowels, which can produce short bursts of pain. Jabs to the ribs can sometimes take your breath away, and punches to the bladder can trigger the release of urine. Fortunately, none of these blows can induce labor or cause complications with your pregnancy. The kicking should settle down toward the end of your pregnancy, when your baby doesn't have as much room to move around.

Why do loud movies cause my baby to move?

❏ a.   Because loud noises hurt his ears.
❏ b.   Because the vibrations from the sound
        waves create bubbles in the amniotic fluid.
❏ c.   Because the baby can hear them.
❏ d.   All of the above.

Answer:

C.

Many pregnant women report that their unborn babies move in response to loud noises. And though it's unlikely your baby is scared or bothered by what's on-screen, he most definitely hears it. By the 28th week, your baby's sense of hearing is fully developed, meaning that anything you're hearing—especially if it's Dolby Digital Sound loud—he's hearing, too. If your baby revs up when you're at the movies, it's most likely that the commotion has woken him from a nap and he's stretching his legs. A sudden jump in your heart rate (say, if you're watching an action or horror film) may get him moving, too. Both are normal and pose no risk to your baby.

True or False:

It is possible for my baby to scratch or poke a hole through the amniotic sac.

Answer:

false.

The amniotic sac lining may look paper thin on an ultrasound, but in fact it's sturdy enough to keep even the strongest baby from poking through. It's also flexible, designed to conform to your baby's every punch, kick, and tumble. And though a baby's nails can grow long by full term, amniotic fluid keeps them soft enough so that he can't scratch himself or your insides. When your sac breaks, it won't be because he clawed his way through it; it will be because you're about to give birth.

#16

What do bruises on my belly indicate?

❑ a.   Your amniotic sac has broken.
❑ b.   You bumped into something.
❑ c.   Your baby kicked you too hard.
❑ d.   You are pregnant with twins.

Answer:
b.

Belly bruising isn't uncommon during pregnancy, especially in the third trimester. During this time, maneuvering with your belly is about as easy as doing the limbo with a watermelon strapped to your torso. You probably bumped into something. As long as it wasn't a hard hit to the abdomen (and you'd remember if it was), a little bruising is nothing to worry about.

The purpling could also be a symptom of your growing tummy. As the baby grows, some of the veins under your skin may move to the surface and rupture, causing bruising. This effect is normal and will go away after you give birth.

Why do some women not have a "baby bump" at 20 weeks, whereas others are huge?

❑ a.   Some babies are smaller than others.

❑ b.   Some women are in better shape, so they don't show as quickly.

❑ c.   Some women's tummies don't stretch as quickly.

❑ d.   All of the above.

Answer:

b.

Generally, women who are in good physical condition during their first pregnancy don't start to show until they're about 20 weeks along. (Second pregnancies usually become notice-able earlier, between 12 and 18 weeks.) If you're sporting a tiny tummy, consider yourself lucky. Once your bump arrives, you'll find that everyday things—sleeping, walking, and getting up from the couch, to name just a few—are much more difficult. Enjoy your svelte-ness while it lasts.

As for those women who look like they're smuggling a basketball, the following factors are usually to blame:

- **Overeating:** Women who eat more calories than they burn tend to gain pregnancy weight too quickly.
- **Multiples:** Women carrying more than one baby are, understandably, going to get bigger, faster.
- **Small frame:** Small or petite women tend to show sooner than women with longer torsos.
- **Bloating:** This condition is common and generally a result of not drinking enough water (counterintuitive, but true). It's also a normal consequence of your sluggish gastrointestinal tract, which slows in response to a surge of the pregnancy-sustaining hormone progesterone.

Do unborn babies poop in the womb?

- ❑ a.   Only if the baby is in distress or overdue.
- ❑ b.   Only if the mother has been eating lots of fiber.
- ❑ c.   Only if there's a problem with the umbilical cord.
- ❑ d.   No, babies poop only after they're born, when there's milk or formula in their stomachs.

Answer:

a.

A baby's first stool, called meconium, is a thick, greenish substance made from various things the baby has swallowed: mucus, bile, intestinal cells, lanugo (the fine hairs on his back that are normally shed before birth), vernix caseosa (a skin secretion), stuff like that. It usually makes its first appearance in your bundle of joy's diaper, but for about 12 percent of babies, it is passed before birth. This happens more frequently in pregnancies that last more than 40 weeks, but it can happen earlier.

Passing meconium before birth may be a sign that the baby is in distress, and thus it is generally considered a medical emergency. Also, potentially fatal respiratory problems can develop if the baby inhales the contaminated amniotic fluid. Babies in the United States rarely die from this condition, known as meconium aspiration syndrome (MAS), since doctors usually induce labor if they suspect meconium has been passed. If, when your water breaks, you notice dark specks in the fluid, call your doctor or get to a hospital as soon as you can.

Can unborn babies feel pain?

❏ a.   No. Human pain receptors don't develop until after birth.

❏ b.   No. The higher intelligence necessary to understand pain doesn't develop until about six months.

❏ c.   Yes, but probably only during the third trimester.

❏ d.   Yes. Pain can be felt as soon as the brain and spinal cord develop, around the fifth week of pregnancy.

Answer:

C.

Scientists believe fetuses can feel pain. But, according to Mark Rosen, an obstetrical anesthesiologist at the University of California at San Francisco and the anesthesiologist for the very first open fetal operation, it doesn't happen before 28 weeks gestation (or your 30th week of pregnancy).

It's a heated debate, since anti-abortion activists have long contended that fetuses can feel pain as early as 18 weeks, and doctors have been pressed to use anesthesia for fetuses during late-term abortions. It is true that as early as 18 weeks, fetuses have been observed recoiling at the touch of a scalpel; however, Rosen attributes this reaction to a reflex, not the sensation of pain.

In 2005, Rosen and his colleagues examined more than 2,000 medical journal articles supporting both sides of the debate. They determined that although fetuses start forming pain receptors as early as 8 weeks, the part of the brain that routes information—which would allow the fetus to feel pain, not just react to it—doesn't form until the third trimester.

Which of these actions is most likely to make your baby kick?

- ❏ a. Jumping up and down 10 times.
- ❏ b. Eating something sweet.
- ❏ c. Running a feather over your belly.
- ❏ d. Chewing on ice.

Answer:

b.

Assuming you're far enough along in your pregnancy to feel your baby's movements (generally between 16 and 22 weeks), there are things you can do to get your baby kicking. Here are just a few:

Eat sugar. First have a fast-burning sugar, such as a glass of orange juice or a candy bar, to wake up your baby. Then eat a slower-burning sugar, such as a bagel or a piece of bread, to keep him awake long enough for you to feel his movements.

Eat spicy food. A piquant dish may also get your little one's juices flowing.

Play music. Place a pair of headphones against your belly and press Play. Unborn babies have been known to perk up at the sound of melodies.

Sit still. Lie down in a quiet room for a while; chances are, you'll feel your baby in no time.

Touch your belly. Some babies will move in response to a jiggle, poke, or pat.

Watch loud movies. Action movies with lots of explosions can get your baby moving.

True or False:

There's no such thing as a baby that's "too active" in the womb.

Answer:
true.

An active baby is a happy baby. It's when she stops moving
that you need to worry.

Every baby is different. Some seem to move all day long;
others move only in response to their mom's activities (eating
sugar and resting after an active day are generally what do it).
Keep in mind that babies move while they're sleeping, too; even
if it feels like yours is always awake, she may not be.

And, by the way, no studies have shown a link between
activity in the womb with activity after birth. So just because
your little one likes to spend all day tumbling around your
belly doesn't mean she'll be a terror as a toddler.

In the womb, babies can see:

❏ a.   Changes in light.

❏ b.   Anything within about 2 inches of their faces.

❏ c.   Nothing. A baby's eyes do not open until after birth.

❏ d.   Nothing. It's too dark in the womb.

Answer:

a.

A fetus's eyes open around 28 weeks gestation, and though we don't know exactly how much they can see, researchers agree that they probably see something. Studies show that from about 30 weeks of pregnancy, if a bright light is shone onto a mother's abdomen, her unborn baby will move away from it.

Most likely, the only thing your little one sees is changes in hue. Basically, his environment looks either dark or, well, darker. Similar to the way we can see light beneath our closed eyelids on a sunny day, a baby can probably see glimmers making their way into the womb.

Whether or not your baby sees anything else—his own hands in front of his face or the umbilical cord floating beside him—is unknown, though studies of twin pregnancies have shown that twins interact before birth, suggesting that they may see each other inside the womb.

True or False:

Babies can cry in the womb.

Answer:
true.

Ultrasound images of infants in the womb suggest that 28-week-old fetuses can silently "cry" in response to a noise stimulus. To investigate, researchers played 90-decibel noises via a speaker placed on the abdomens of pregnant women and recorded the responses using an ultrasound scan. What they found was a visible reaction that resembled that of an infant crying. "Even the bottom lip quivers," lead pediatrician Ed Mitchell told reporters.

On the other hand, babies can't cry out loud until they're born. In the womb, babies are totally immersed in amniotic fluid, so there is no air in the lungs with which to produce sounds. It is only after they're born that the lungs can fully expand to take in air and let out those first miraculous shrieks.

True or False:

How much you eat can determine the sex of your baby.

Answer:

true.

It's not a hard-and-fast rule, but research has shown that women who consume fewer calories at the time of conception are more likely to conceive girls than women with heartier appetites.

According to a study conducted by the universities of Exeter and Oxford, women with higher total daily calorie intakes were more likely to give birth to sons than women who skimped on meals. Exactly *what* you eat at the time of conception may also have some bearing on your baby's gender. The study, which surveyed 740 new moms, found that potassium-rich diets tipped the gender scales toward boy babies. There was also an association between eating breakfast cereals and having sons, though it was unclear whether that was related to the extra calories or to the cereal itself.

But don't start skimping or splurging on meals. The study found no cause-and-effect relationship when it came to women's diets and their babies' genders; it only found associations. Most experts would still agree that your chances of having either gender is still, basically, 50-50.

What happens if I take a really hot bath?

❏ a.   Your muscles will relax, which can cause the uterus to contract and potentially trigger preterm labor.

❏ b.   Your body temperature will rise, which can decrease blood flow to your baby.

❏ c.   Your body will stop producing the hormones needed to sustain your pregnancy.

❏ d.   Your baby will grow faster.

Answer:

b.

You can take a bath, but keep the water temperature below 100°F. Any hotter and you could overheat, which might increase your heart rate and decrease blood flow. That could place stress on your baby and potentially damage fetal cells.

Since we're on the topic, you should also avoid doing anything that significantly raises your body temperature. That means no hot tubs, electric blankets, saunas, steam showers, or exercising in hot weather. Hot showers are fine because, unlike baths, your entire body isn't submerged.

Always be on the lookout for these signs of overheating: dizziness or faintness, chills, extreme thirst, nausea.

Extreme temperatures are particularly dangerous during the first trimester, when the baby's major organs are developing. If you want to be extra careful, stay out of the tub until you're past your 14th week.

If you've already taken a dip in a hot tub without realizing the danger, don't panic. Studies show that most women get out of a hot tub before their body temperatures reach dangerous levels, simply because they get uncomfortable. If you didn't, or if you're still worried, talk to your doctor.

Can I use bubble bath, bath salts, or bath oils?

❑ a.   No, the ingredients can degrade your baby's amniotic sac.

❑ b.   No, the ingredients can enter the blood-stream, where they can possibly cause birth defects or other complications.

❑ c.   No, the ingredients may irritate your skin and vaginal area.

❑ d.   Yes, it's fine to use these products while you're pregnant.

Answer:

C.

As long as your cervix is closed and your membranes aren't ruptured (as is usually the case until you're nearing labor), there is no danger of these products reaching your baby.

But bubble baths may present other problems. Some bath solutions can upset the vagina's pH balance, which in turn lessens the "good" bacteria growing there and allows the "bad" bacteria to thrive. This imbalance causes vaginal infections, whose symptoms include irritation, discharge, and odor. It also carries an increased risk of bladder infections, since a more sensitive vaginal area can increase the risk of bacteria moving into the bladder. Some doctors recommend emptying the bladder before and after a bubble bath to lessen the chance of infection.

Oh, and one other thing: Some women's skin becomes more sensitive during pregnancy. The bath salts, oils, or bubbles that used to leave your skin smooth and sexy may now cause rashes and irritation. To lessen this risk, try using a bath solution made for sensitive skin. Or just skip the bubbles altogether.

#27

Why is massage not recommended during the first trimester?

❑ a.   Massage can release toxins in the body, which can cause developmental problems for your baby during this most fragile time.

❑ b.   You may lose consciousness.

❑ c.   Massage therapists can charge more for massages done later in pregnancy.

❑ d.   Massage therapists don't want to be held responsible if you have a miscarriage.

Answer:

d.

Though it's true that rubbing particular body areas—namely, ankles and wrists—can trigger uterine contractions, massage during pregnancy is unlikely to cause problems, especially if given by a practitioner familiar with prenatal therapy.

Still, most therapists and spas offer tailored pregnancy massages only after the first trimester. The reason is because it is during this time that most miscarriages occur. If a pregnant woman miscarries in the days after a massage, the loss could be blamed on the therapist (even though the miscarriage likely would have happened anyway). So be sure to tell your therapist or the spa receptionists that you're expecting.

Massage during pregnancy offers many benefits, including reduced anxiety, relief from muscle aches and joint pain, reduced swelling, and improved circulation. It's not recommended for women with a high-risk pregnancy; preeclampsia (pregnancy-induced hypertension); severe swelling, high blood pressure, sudden severe headaches, or unusual bleeding.

The only other point to keep in mind is your own comfort. If you're prone to nausea, you may want to ask the therapist to skip the scented oils.

#28

Is it safe to have a foot massage?

❑ a.   No, regular foot massages increase the risk that your baby will be in breech (foot-first) position when you go into labor.

❑ b.   Probably, but pressure points on the foot can trigger uterine contractions.

❑ c.   No, massaging the feet can release feel-good hormones in your body, which can alter your baby's brain chemistry.

❑ d.   Yes, foot massage is harmless during pregnancy.

Answer:

b.

Though it's unlikely that a simple kneading of the feet will do any damage, there are pressure points—specifically, on the ankles and the inside of the heel—that, when rubbed a certain way, can cause uterine contractions. Theoretically, these contractions can jump-start labor or trigger a miscarriage. But unless your massage therapist is well versed in the ways of acupressure, it's highly unlikely that a little rubbing of these areas will do more than cause a tremble in your uterine walls.

Gentle massage, even around these sensitive areas, is fine. In fact, a foot massage while you're pregnant is a great way to reduce stress and fight fatigue. Your feet are working hard carrying all your growing weight. They deserve a good rub!

29

What skin-care products should I avoid?

❏ a. Certain anti-aging creams and cosmetics.
❏ b. Hemorrhoid creams.
❏ c. All products containing blue dyes.
❏ d. All products containing a sun block.

Answer:

a.

Since everything you put in—and on—your body can potentially affect your baby, it's good to know what you're slathering on your skin. Most makeup and skin creams are safe; however, a few have been linked to birth defects or may adversely affect the mother and should be used with caution. These include

- Retinoids (also known as Accutane, Differin, Retin-A, Renova, tretinoin, retinoic acid, retinol, retinyl linoleate, retinyl palmitate, Tazorac, and Avage), used for preventing acne and wrinkles
- Salicylic acid, used to treat acne
- Beta hydroxy acid (BHA), a form of salicylic acid used in some exfoliants to treat wrinkles
- Self-tanners, which haven't been proved safe for use during pregnancy
- Hair-removal products, which may cause more irritation than they did before you were pregnant
- Soy-based products (including lecithin, phosphatidylcholine, and textured vegetable protein), which may darken the skin and worsen the so-called mask of pregnancy. (Note that products containing "active soy" do not have this effect.)

30

Is it dangerous to get a bikini wax?

❏ a. Yes, the heat of the wax can raise your body temperature, which can be dangerous for your baby.

❏ b. Yes, the chemicals in the wax can cause birth defects.

❏ c. Not really, but pregnancy makes your skin extra sensitive, so waxing will really hurt.

❏ d. No, but you need pubic hair to keep your uterus warm.

Answer:

C.

A bikini wax won't hurt your baby, but it'll probably hurt you, thanks to the increased blood flow to the surface of your skin that can make you more sensitive (especially down there). Therefore, your usual waxing sessions are going to be a lot more painful than they used to be, and you'll likely have more skin irritation and broken blood vessels. To alleviate these problems, estheticians may use "hard," or "cold," wax, which is gentler on the skin.

When it comes to your baby, the main concern is the possibility of infection, from either nonsterile conditions or tiny skin abrasions from the waxing. Be sure that the facility is clean and that the esthetician uses a fresh bowl of wax (and doesn't "double dip," which can introduce bacteria into the pot). Afterward, thoroughly clean the area with warm soap and water until the redness and irritation are relieved.

31

Is it okay to burn scented candles?

❏ a.   No, because certain scents may trigger miscarriages.

❏ b.   Yes, but you may not be able to smell them anymore.

❏ c.   Yes, but they may aggravate your allergies or make you feel sick.

❏ d.   No, the chemicals can harm your baby.

Answer:

C.

Certain smells may make you nauseous now that you've got an extra-sensitive sniffer (though fragrances that mimic sweet foods are less likely to do so). In addition, since allergies and asthma are sometimes exacerbated by pregnancy, your longtime favorite candles may begin to trigger an allergic reaction, such as itchy eyes and a runny nose. This may be due to the fragrance itself or to the small particulates released into the air when the candle burns. Burning scented candles can also contribute to poor indoor air quality, according to the U.S. Environmental Protection Agency. To keep the air clear, follow these tips:

- Use beeswax or soy (instead of paraffin wax) candles.
- Avoid multiple-wick candles.
- Trim the wick to ¼ inch before lighting.
- Keep your candle in a draft-free area to maintain a low, steady flame.
- Throw away candles that leave a sooty residue.
- Increase ventilation in rooms where candles are burning.
- Don't burn candles for more than an hour.
- Make sure the wick is lead-free. Lead has been banned from U.S.-made candles since 2003; double-check those purchased before that date or made in another country.

32

Can I color my hair?

❏ a.   Only if you're going from light to dark.
❏ b.   Only if you're going from dark to light.
❏ c.   Yes, but make sure to deep-condition
           afterward, since pregnancy makes your
           hair extra dry.
❏ d.   Yes, but wait until after your first
           trimester.

Answer:
d.

Most doctors agree that the occasional touch-up should be safe, though some advise waiting until after the first trimester when the baby's major organs have developed. But spending every day around dyes may be a little riskier. A Swedish study conducted between 1973 and 1994 found that hairdressers were slightly more likely to have babies born small or with major birth defects such as heart defects, cleft palate or lip, and spina bifida. These results may be due to other factors, such as the prolonged standing and bending required of the job. Play it safe, by following these precautions:

- Wear gloves to minimize contact with dye.
- Work in a well-ventilated room to minimize fumes.
- Don't leave dye on longer than recommended.
- Consider highlights. When applied correctly, the dye doesn't touch the scalp, so you won't absorb chemicals.
- Use all-natural vegetable dye or henna.

If you do dye your hair, don't be surprised if the color isn't exactly what you expected. Hormonal changes during pregnancy may cause your hair to react differently to chemicals. And since your hair grows faster when you're pregnant, you may need more frequent touch-ups.

33

Can I use self-tanning creams?

❑ a.   No, because self-tanners can alter your baby's skin.

❑ b.   No, because self-tanners contain ingredients that haven't been thoroughly studied.

❑ c.   Yes, as long as you don't use them more than once a week.

❑ d.   Yes, but they may turn your skin a different color than you hoped for.

Answer:

b.

It's unlikely that self-tanners will cause problems, but these products haven't been tested enough to know for sure what harm they might do. To be safe, you may want to avoid the fake bake until after your baby is born.

Don't go rushing poolside, either. UV rays may prevent your body from absorbing folic acid, which is essential for helping with the development of your baby's brain and spinal cord. In addition, when you're pregnant your skin is especially sensitive, so even a little time in the sun can cause a burn.

Your best bet? Stay natural or invest in a good bronzer—and save (safe) tanning for when you're a mom.

#34

Is having my teeth professionally whitened a bad idea?

- ❏ a.   It's fine, but your teeth may be more prone to cavities afterward.
- ❏ b.   No, but your teeth may not whiten much.
- ❏ c.   Yes, there's a chance that the chemicals may interfere with your baby's development.
- ❏ d.   You can try, but your mommy-to-be saliva contains protective enzymes that make teeth whiteners ineffective.

Answer:

C.

Not enough studies have been undertaken to determine whether the peroxide used in teeth whitening is harmful to a developing fetus. Consequently, most doctors advise women to postpone treatment until their babies are born. Whitening toothpastes are fine. Just make sure you find one that contains fluoride, since pregnancy also makes you more prone to tooth decay and gum disease.

If you do decide to whiten your teeth professionally, be prepared for a bit of discomfort. Hormonal changes during pregnancy can cause sore and swollen gums, and the chemicals in teeth whiteners may aggravate these symptoms. Your teeth may also be more sensitive after the procedure.

35

What are the pitfalls of wearing high heels while I'm pregnant?

❏ a.   They can cause vertigo.
❏ b.   They can make your feet swell.
❏ c.   They can increase your risk for blood clots.
❏ d.   There are none. In fact, heels may
            strengthen your pelvic muscles in
            preparation for labor.

Answer:
b.

During pregnancy, your heart pumps about 50 percent more blood and other fluids through your body to nourish your growing baby. This extra fluid can cause swelling of the hands, feet, ankles, and legs—all of which can be worsened by walking on tiptoe all day (essentially what you're doing when wearing high heels).

If your feet aren't yet swollen, it's a safe bet that cramming your piggies into a pair of Jimmy Choos will do the trick. Wearing high heels can also exacerbate the usual pregnancy-related back pains.

Another reason to steer clear of stilettos: You may fall. As your belly grows and your center of gravity changes, common activities like walking become more and more difficult. Stick with flats until your baby's born.

There is one exception (besides a really important date night): Wearing moderately high heels may ease symptoms of sciatica. If you're suffering from this painful nerve condition, a pair of pumps might help.

36

Can a genital or belly piercing complicate a pregnancy?

❏ a.   Any unhealed piercing could cause an infection, which could trigger early labor.

❏ b.   A nipple piercing could stimulate uterine contractions.

❏ c.   A labia piercing could make your vagina more likely to tear during childbirth.

❏ d.   A navel piercing could affect the way your belly stretches as your baby grows.

Answer:

a.

Any completely healed piercing should be safe; however, you might want to switch to polytetrafluoroethylene jewelry (the flexible plastic used for surgical implants), which will be more comfortable, until you deliver. Also, to keep the holes from closing, you can replace jewelry with clean fishing line.

If you have a new piercing that's not completely healed, watch to ensure it doesn't become infected. New piercings are more prone to infections, which could potentially affect your baby or even trigger early labor. Call your doctor if, around the site of your piercing, you notice any redness, swelling, warmth, pus, or pain.

If you have vaginal piercings, remove all jewelry from them when you go into labor. And know that the site of your piercing may be torn or stretched during childbirth. Same goes for belly or nipple piercings, both of which will stretch as you get bigger.

37

Why is Botox unsafe for use during pregnancy?

- ❑ a.   It could cause birth defects.
- ❑ b.   It could cause a miscarriage.
- ❑ c.   You might be more sensitive to its effects.
- ❑ d.   All of the above.

d.

According to its manufacturers, Botox is not recommended for pregnant women and breastfeeding mothers. Let's not forget: The "tox" stands for "toxin." In small amounts, this toxin works to paralyze muscles; hence the smoothed-over look of your smile and frown lines after an injection. In large amounts, it can cause serious illness and even death.

Though the amount used for cosmetic and medical procedures has been deemed safe for the general population, no studies have been undertaken to determine whether it affects a growing fetus. But animal studies don't bode well: Tests on pregnant rats showed a link between high levels of Botox and low birth weights as well as problems with fetal bone development. Pregnant rabbits given high doses of the toxin experienced miscarriages and had babies with birth defects. Granted, the doses administered in these tests were much higher, proportionally, than those that would ever be used on people. Nonetheless, doctors advise that women wait until they have given birth and finished breastfeeding before getting an injection.

On the upside, your skin de-wrinkles during pregnancy, thanks to water retention, increased blood flow, and added hormones. So you'll be naturally (not chemically) radiant.

#38

Why are my nipples turning brown and getting huge?

❏ a.　　They're getting bigger and darker so your newborn can easily find them.

❏ b.　　Your hormones are darkening your skin, and not just in the nipples.

❏ c.　　The nipples are stretching because your breasts are growing.

❏ d.　　All of the above.

Answer:

d.

During pregnancy, the already darkened areas of the skin (moles, freckles, areolae, nipples, and the faint line that runs from the center of the pelvis to the belly button) darken further thanks to an increase in progesterone pumping through your body. It's unclear what the purpose of this skin darkening is, but most doctors agree it helps poor-sighted newborns find the nipple.

Most of these changes will return to normal a few months after you give birth, though there's a chance your nipples won't revert completely to their prepregnancy hue.

As for nipple size, they're growing because your breasts are growing. During pregnancy, breasts often grow by at least a cup size, which also stretches the nipple. Once you're no longer breastfeeding, your breasts and nipples should return to their normal size (though some women say their nipples remain slightly enlarged).

Why is hair growing around my belly button?

❑ a.   Pregnancy hormones cause hair to darken and become more noticeable.

❑ b.   Your baby's kicks stimulate hair follicles.

❑ c.   Pregnancy hormones sprout hair in all sorts of unexpected places.

❑ d.   Hair was already growing there, you just didn't notice it until your belly got so big.

Answer:

C.

Pregnancy introduces all sorts of new hair-related issues. Basically, you'll have more of it in more places. These hair-growth patterns are the result of increased hormones pumping through your body. It's temporary, usually starting in the first trimester and continuing throughout your ninth month.

In addition to new hairs around your belly button, you may also notice unusual growth patterns on your face, breasts, arms, legs, and back. If your new hirsute state bothers you, feel free to tweeze or wax; just don't use chemical hair removers since they have not been sufficiently tested for use by pregnant women. And know that depilatories may be more painful to your more-sensitive-than-usual skin.

40

Will my belly button stay an "outie" once the baby is born?

❑ a. Yes, that's why all moms have "outies."

❑ b. No, but there are over-the-counter belly button creams that can reverse the change.

❑ c. No, your belly button will return to its old self after your baby is born.

❑ d. It's different for everyone.

Answer:

d.

As your belly grows, your belly button, which is tethered to the abdominal wall from the inside, pushes out. For some women, the resulting change in shape is slight; for others, the belly button pops out so much that it shows through clothing.

Like most physical changes that occur during pregnancy, this too shall pass. Your belly button should return to its mostly normal—albeit slightly stretched—state after you give birth. For a few women, a pregnancy-induced outie will stay that way. If it really bothers you, plastic surgeons can resculpt the navel in a procedure called an umbilicoplasty.

41

What will pregnancy do to my breast implants?

❏ a.   A growing belly might cause them to shift.

❏ b.   Nothing. The breasts will enlarge naturally.

❏ c.   The implants may prevent breasts from growing as they naturally would during pregnancy.

❏ d.   The body may break down the implants as it readies the breasts for milk production.

Answer:

b.

Implants or no implants, your breasts are going to get bigger
as your belly grows. This increase is caused by water retention,
added fat, and the maturing of milk glands. It will in no way
affect the placement or constitution of implants.

In fact, implants may offer some perks (no pun intended).
The loss of volume and shape—aka "saggy breasts"—associated
with pregnancy and breast-feeding is less dramatic in women
with implants, probably because the implants don't lose any
of their original volume or shape. Implants won't spare you
entirely from the postchildbirth sag, but they will make it less
noticeable.

42

Why can pregnancy make naturally curly hair suddenly straight?

❏ a.　　Pregnancy hormones affect hair and skin.

❏ b.　　Dehydration, which is common during pregnancy, can leave locks limp and lifeless.

❏ c.　　Your body is diverting all nutrients toward nourishing your baby, causing changes in the way hair grows.

❏ d.　　Your hair is just too tired to curl.

Answer:

a.

The hormones required to grow and incubate a fetus are a potent brew, and a nine-month-long bad-hair day is just one in the litany of physical changes they'll set off—and that you'll have to embrace. Some women notice their hair getting darker or lighter; some see their pin-straight tresses start to curl; and others find that their normally curly locks go limp.

Your mane will likely return to its prepregnancy state once your baby is born; but for a small number of women, the change is permanent. If that happens, try to enjoy your new-found 'do. If you want to get a perm to restore your ringlets, it's probably safe to do so; however, most hairdressers will recommend that you wait until after you give birth, since pregnancy hormones may make your hair react differently to the chemicals.

43

True or False:

You can still have your period while pregnant.

Answer:
false.

Bleeding or spotting during pregnancy is common, occurring in nearly 30 percent of pregnant women, but it's not indicative of a menstrual period. It is most often caused by the following:

- **Implantation:** As the fertilized egg burrows into the uterine lining, you may notice light bleeding around the time when your next period would normally be due. Implantation bleeding lasts only a day or two and is usually much lighter than a regular period.

- **Infections:** Yeast infections, bacterial vaginosis, and sexually transmitted infections can irritate the cervix and cause spotting, especially after sex or a vaginal exam.

- **Intercourse:** During pregnancy, the cervix is tender and sensitive, which can cause light bleeding after sex. It's worth mentioning to your doctor since it could be caused by placenta previa, a somewhat rare condition in which the placenta partially or completely blocks the cervix.

Bleeding could also be a sign of more serious conditions, including ectopic pregnancy (when the fertilized egg implants outside the uterus), placental problems, or miscarriage. To be safe, call your doctor if you notice any spotting, especially if accompanied by pain or cramping.

44

Why does my pee smell weird?

- ❏ a.   Your baby's waste empties into your bladder.
- ❏ b.   Hormonal changes affect body odor.
- ❏ c.   You're peeing so frequently that the urine doesn't have time to lose its odor.
- ❏ d.   You may have a sexually transmitted infection.

Answer:
b.

If you haven't already noticed, the hormones needed to grow your baby do quite a bit more than that. Sadly, the changes include making your pee smell a little funky. And these days your urine isn't the only thing that may stink. Increased hormones may also affect the smell of your body and vaginal area. It's embarrassing, but temporary. You'll return to your prepregnancy aromas once the baby is born. For now, all you can do is shower. Don't use vaginal douches or intimate deodorant, both of which could cause other problems.

Keep in mind, though, that your changing scent could be caused by more than mere hormones. Foul-smelling urine may be a sign of a urinary tract infection. UTIs are more common during pregnancy, since the uterus sits directly on the bladder, which can inhibit urine flow and promote infection. When in doubt, call your doctor. If treated, urinary infections pose little risk to the fetus; untreated, they can lead to kidney problems, which can cause early labor and low birth weight.

45

Why does my mouth feel so dry?

❏ a.   You're probably dehydrated.

❏ b.   Your salivary glands don't work as well during pregnancy.

❏ c.   You're peeing so much that your body is losing fluids.

❏ d.   It's not; your brain only tells you it is so that you drink enough water to nourish your baby.

Answer:

a.

During pregnancy, your body pumps about 50 percent more blood and other fluids through your body, which can leave you dehydrated and perpetually thirsty. So drink up and avoid the host of problems triggered by dehydration, from dry mouth, headaches, and nausea to cramps, swelling, and potentially preterm labor. Doctors recommend that pregnant women drink 10 to 12 glasses a day, and more if you exercise or spend time outside in hot weather.

If you can't seem to lose the cotton mouth, hard candy and sugarless gum may help get your salivary glands working again.

46

Does vaginal massage offer benefits during pregnancy?

❑ a.   No. There is no benefit. In fact, it might introduce bacteria into the uterus.

❑ b.   Yes. It can intensify your orgasms.

❑ c.   Daily vaginal massages may prevent tearing during childbirth.

❑ d.   Vaginal massages will make childbirth less painful, but only if they're done while you're in labor.

Answer:

C.

Perineal massage—stretching the skin between the vagina and the anus—has long been suggested as a way to prevent tearing and avoid episiotomies during childbirth. Some studies have shown it to be effective; others indicate no benefits. But it certainly can't hurt. (Note: Women with active herpes lesions should not do perineal massage.) Proponents recommend starting around the 34th week and doing daily massages until your due date. Here's how:

1. After bathing, sit or lie down on a clean towel.

2. Apply a generous amount of lubricant (try vitamin E oil) to your hands and around your perineum (the area between your vagina and anus). Put both thumbs about one or two inches into your vagina.

3. Press down, firmly but gently, toward the anus and outward toward your thighs until you feel a stretch. You should feel pressure, stinging, or discomfort, but it shouldn't hurt. Hold this position for several minutes.

4. Move your thumbs back and forth along the sides of your vagina, avoiding the urinary opening, for three or four more minutes.

47

Why do my farts smell so bad during pregnancy?

❏ a.   Changes in your diet can upset your digestive tract.

❏ b.   Your pregnant body digests its meals more slowly than normal, giving food more time in the intestines to ferment and cause smelly gas.

❏ c.   They don't smell any worse than usual; your nose is just more sensitive.

❏ d.   Your body is processing more waste.

Answer:

b.

Pregnancy relaxes the muscles in your digestive tract, which in turn slows digestion and results in constipation, bloating, burping, and gas. The longer food stays in your intestines, the more time it has to ferment and produce bacteria. And bacteria smells.

There isn't much you can do to eliminate the problem, but try these tips to make it a bit less bothersome.

- **Avoid "farty" foods:** Onions, beans, cabbage, radishes, prunes, apricots, cauliflower, broccoli, and Brussels sprouts can all make you gassy, as can carbonated beverages.
- **Nix the milk:** Dairy products make some people cut the cheese. If you reduce your intake, be sure to get calcium from other sources—you need it to help build your baby's bones.
- **Chew food slowly and thoroughly:** That way, you'll swallow less air as you eat.
- **Stop chewing gum:** You swallow more air than normal when chewing gum, and that excess air can lead to farting.
- **Eat several small meals instead of one big meal:** This allows you to digest food before gas builds up.
- **Take a stool softener:** Constipation causes gas, so treating it may help reduce excess wind.

#48

Why am I snoring more now that I'm pregnant?

- ❑ a. You aren't sleeping as soundly as you used to, which causes snoring.
- ❑ b. Pregnancy makes the mucous membranes in your nose and throat swell, which causes snoring.
- ❑ c. The added poundage of pregnancy causes snoring.
- ❑ d. You're breathing for two, and snoring helps you take in more oxygen.

Answer:

b.

During pregnancy, the mucous membranes in your nose and throat thicken and swell as a result of both hormones and increased blood flow. These blocked nasal passages keep you snoring at night and stuffy by day. Some women also experience frequent nosebleeds during pregnancy.

It's all normal and temporary. Pregnancy-induced stuffiness should go away once your baby is born. Until then, try using a saline nasal spray before bed, drinking plenty of water, and running a humidifier in your bedroom. Adhesive nose strips may also facilitate breathing.

49

Why do I often feel bloated and gassy?

❏ a.   Your baby is gassy.
❏ b.   It helps stretch out your skin so your belly can grow.
❏ c.   You've been eating too much.
❏ d.   Pregnancy slows your digestion, which makes you gassy.

Answer:
d.

Bloating is common during pregnancy, thanks to increased levels of progesterone working to relax the muscles of your gastrointestinal tract. This relaxation slows your digestive process, which leads to gas, constipation, and bloating. On the upside, sluggish digestion gives nutrients from your food extra time to enter your bloodstream and nourish your baby.

Try the following to alleviate bloating:

- Take a stool softener daily.
- Drink plenty of water, and avoid carbonated beverages.
- Eat smaller meals throughout the day.
- Chew food thoroughly.
- Avoid foods such as Brussels sprouts, cabbage, asparagus, beans, cauliflower, and anything fried or especially fatty.
- Sit up straight while eating so that your stomach has room to work.
- Take a short walk after meals to stimulate digestion.
- Take an over-the-counter gas remedy containing simethicone.

Call your doctor if your abdominal pain is only on one side or accompanied by sudden nausea and vomiting, bleeding, or diarrhea. These could be due to more than just mere gas pains.

50

Is it dangerous to sleep on my stomach?

❏ a.　　No, but you won't be comfortable that way for long.

❏ b.　　Yes, it could compress the uterus and inhibit your baby's growth.

❏ c.　　Yes, it could deprive your baby of oxygen.

❏ d.　　Yes, it could cut off circulation to your legs.

Answer:

a.

Sleeping on your stomach won't hurt your baby, but by about the fourth or fifth month, your bulging belly will be too much of an obstacle for it to be comfortable. Ever try sleeping on top of a basketball? Now's your chance.

The best position to sleep in during pregnancy is on the left side. This position optimizes the flow of blood and nutrients to the uterus by keeping the baby's weight off the major veins that bring blood back to the heart. It also keeps the uterus off any of your major organs (including the liver, which is on the right side).

If you have trouble staying sideways, try propping a pillow between your knees and lying with your legs slightly bent. You can also buy a full-body pillow, which can help you stay propped on your side all night long.

#51

Can severe constipation harm my baby?

❏ a.   If there's enough of it, compacted stool
       can press against your baby and restrict
       growth.
❏ b.   If there's enough of it, compacted stool can
       restrict your baby's movements.
❏ c.   Stagnant poop can release toxins into your
       bloodstream, which can harm your baby.
❏ d.   Constipation can't hurt your baby, but it
       can hurt you.

Answer:

d.

More than half of all pregnant women suffer from constipation, caused by the progesterone-induced slowing of the digestive process necessary for your baby to receive proper nourishment. Here are some things you can do to stay regular:

- Eat lots of fiber, from foods such as whole-grain bread and fresh fruits and vegetables.
- Drink plenty of water, at least 10 to 12 glasses a day.
- Exercise, which can stimulate a sluggish digestive process.
- Take a stool softener containing simethicone daily (some prenatal vitamins already contain this agent).
- Reduce or eliminate iron supplements; too much iron can worsen constipation. You can consume sufficient levels of iron through your diet or regular prenatal vitamin.

During bowel movements, try not to push too hard; this may irritate the cervix, which could cause minor bleeding (spotting). It isn't dangerous to your baby, but it can be disconcerting. Persistent pushing can also cause hemorrhoids, which can hurt. Contact your doctor if you experience constipation accompanied by abdominal pain or alternating diarrhea, since these symptoms could be a sign of something more serious.

52

Why do my nipples sometimes feel like they're burning?

❏ a.   Your breasts are starting to produce milk.

❏ b.   Your breasts are growing, which causes a burning sensation.

❏ c.   More blood is flowing to the breasts, which makes them more sensitive.

❏ d.   Your bra is too tight.

Answer:

C.

As with so many symptoms of pregnancy, you can blame your hormones for this one. Increased levels of estrogen and progesterone send more blood to the breasts, making them sensitive to the touch. Consequently, burning, itching, tender, and throbbing nipples are all common pregnancy complaints.

You'll also notice that your breasts are growing and your areolae are darkening. These are all good signs that your body is readying itself to be a mom.

You can take acetaminophen (Tylenol) if the burning really bothers you. Also, wear a comfortable bra (cotton is best) or go braless, since clothes rubbing against your breasts may aggravate the pain. Keeping your surroundings warm may also help because the burning sensation may intensify when your nipples harden or get cold.

53

Why does it hurt so much to get out of bed?

❑ a.   Your baby is weighing you down.

❑ b.   Since sleep is so important during pregnancy, this pain is your body's way of telling you to stay in bed.

❑ c.   You probably pulled an abdominal muscle.

❑ d.   The ligaments supporting your uterus are being stretched.

Answer:

d.

What you're feeling is round ligament pain, characterized as a brief stabbing sensation or dull ache of the lower abdomen or groin. It happens when the round ligaments (the ligaments surrounding your uterus) stretch and thicken to accommodate pregnancy.

Round ligament pain is most common in the second and third trimesters and generally occurs when you change positions suddenly, such as rolling over in bed or getting up from a sitting or sleeping position. Coughing or laughing can also trigger the pain.

So how can you get yourself out of bed without wincing? Do it slowly. Roll over onto your side, swing your feet over the bed, and slowly use your arms to lift yourself up to a sitting position. Then stand.

If you're having abdominal pain at other times—or if the pain is accompanied by severe cramping, bleeding, fever, or chills—consult your doctor right away. It could be a sign of something more serious, including an ectopic pregnancy.

54

Is it OK to hold in my pee?

❏ a.   No, resisting the urge to pee may force your overfilled bladder to press against your baby.

❏ b.   No, holding it can cause an infection.

❏ c.   You can hold it, but not more than once a day.

❏ d.   You should hold it. In fact, doing so can strengthen the bladder muscles.

Answer:

b.

Go if you've gotta go.

When urine remains too long in your bladder, bacteria will grow and increase your risk of developing a urinary tract infection. UTIs are common during pregnancy because your bladder is compressed and under constant pressure from your growing uterus. Though they're common, they should still be treated promptly. Left untreated, UTIs can lead to kidney infections, which can cause problems for you and your baby.

Another reason against holding it: An inflamed bladder may irritate the uterus and cause contractions, which could potentially trigger preterm labor.

55

Why does pregnancy make me feel itchy?

❏ a.   Your body may be having an allergic reaction to your pregnancy.
❏ b.   Your skin is stretching.
❏ c.   When you're pregnant, your skin can't properly regulate temperature.
❏ d.   You may be in labor.

Answer:

b.

Itchiness is a common pregnancy complaint. It mostly affects the abdomen and breasts, where skin is stretching and tightening. Hormonal changes may aggravate the problem. To alleviate the itching:

- Avoid hot showers; take warm oatmeal baths instead.
- Slather on plenty of unscented moisturizer (some fragrances can further irritate your skin).
- Drink 10 to 12 glasses of water a day.
- Use mild soaps to cleanse your skin.

If the itchiness is unbearable, contact your doctor. Some itchiness is normal, but severe itching of the hands and feet or itchiness accompanied by nausea, vomiting, light-colored stool, fatigue, and a yellowing of the skin can be a sign of cholestasis, a common liver disease that occurs only during pregnancy. Cholestasis can cause fetal distress and preterm birth.

Other causes of itchiness include prurigo, a safe but annoying rash of small red bumps; pruritic urticarial papules and plaques of pregnancy (PUPPP), a similiarly nonthreatening rash that usually begins on the belly and may spread to the rest of the body; and adverse reactions to skin-care products.

56

True or False:

Underwire bras should not be worn during pregnancy because they can inhibit breast growth.

Answer:
false.

It's perfectly fine to sport underwire bras during pregnancy. Assuming it fits correctly, an underwire bra does not inhibit the growth of breast tissue during pregnancy. Plus, as your breasts get bigger—and they will—you may find that you need the added support.

That said, wires beneath your breasts may be uncomfortable, particularly in your third trimester, when your belly swells to just below your rib cage. An underwire may dig into the top of your belly every time you sit down.

Try wearing a supportive wireless bra (like a sports bra) and consider stocking up on nursing bras, which you're going to need should you decide to breast-feed. Since underwires can potentially lead to clogged ducts during breast-feeding, most nursing bras don't have them.

Whichever type of bra you choose, buy them in a few different sizes. Your breasts will change a lot throughout your pregnancy, and some women say they need a different bra for every trimester.

#57

Can the flu affect my unborn baby?

❏ a.   No, the flu is more dangerous for you than
        it is for your baby.

❏ b.   No, you and your baby are protected from
        the flu by your immune system, which is
        stronger when you're pregnant.

❏ c.   Yes, your baby may be born with an even
        more severe form of the flu.

❏ d.   Yes, your baby may contract the flu from
        you through the umbilical cord.

Answer:

a.

Pregnancy weakens your immune system, leaving you more vulnerable not only to catching the flu but also to developing complications from it. It also lessens heart and lung function, which puts you at greater risk for developing pneumonia, a common complication.

Your baby won't catch the flu from you, but that doesn't mean it isn't dangerous to him. Studies have linked sustained high fevers in mothers, particularly during weeks 3 and 7, to birth defects. If you're running a high temperature, take immediate measures to lower it: Soak in a cool bath, sip cold drinks, try to stay hydrated, and take acetaminophen (it's safe during pregnancy). And call your doctor. Certain flu medications are fine to take during pregnancy, especially if the benefit outweighs the risk.

If you haven't yet gotten the flu, now's the time to get vaccinated. Doctors recommend that all pregnant women receive a flu shot at the start of flu season. The shots are safe during pregnancy unless you've had a past adverse reaction to one or are allergic to eggs.

#58

Can severe coughing hurt my baby?

❏ a.   Yes, it could trigger a miscarriage or early labor.
❏ b.   It can deprive the baby of oxygen.
❏ c.   It can damage your baby's hearing.
❏ d.   No. Coughing won't hurt your baby.

Answer:

d.

You can't cough yourself into labor, nor can coughing trigger a miscarriage. Your stomach hurts because you're clenching your abdominal muscles. Although such scrunching can't hurt your baby, it can leave your tummy feeling like you've just done a few too many sit-ups.

To alleviate symptoms, try sucking on cough drops and drinking extra fluids to thin out the mucous secretions that cause coughing. If these remedies don't work, cough medicines such as Mucinex or Robitussin are safe to take—just check with your doctor first. Avoid cold remedies that contain alcohol, and don't ingest decongestants containing pseudoephedrine or phenylephrine, both of which can affect blood flow to the placenta. If your cough is accompanied by a fever or sore throat, call your doctor. You may have strep throat or a sinus infection, which are treatable with antibiotics.

59

Can a yeast infection be passed on to my baby?

❏ a.   Only if the baby comes into contact with
         the yeast during delivery.
❏ b.   Only if the infection goes untreated.
❏ c.   Only if you're in your first trimester. After
         that, the baby is protected by the placenta.
❏ d.   No, yeast infections affect only adults.

Answer:

a.

Thanks to hormonal changes, yeast infections are more common during pregnancy than at any other time in a woman's life. Symptoms include thick white or light yellow discharge that may smell yeasty (like bread); redness, irritation, or itching around the vagina; and burning during urination or intercourse.

A baby can contract a yeast infection during a vaginal delivery. He may develop a yeast infection of the mouth, called thrush, which is easily treated with medication.

Treat your yeast infection with over-the-counter creams and suppositories. To prevent recurring infections:

- Wear breathable clothing and cotton underwear.
- After bathing, dry your vaginal area completely.
- Wipe front to back after urinating or bowel movements.
- Avoid sitting around in damp garments.
- Don't douche or use feminine hygiene sprays; these can upset your vagina's pH balance.
- Eat yogurt or take acidophilus daily.
- Limit your intake of sugar, which encourages the growth of yeast.

See your doctor before starting treatment to make sure you're battling a yeast infection and not something else.

60

True or False:

If I have asthma,
my baby may not be
getting enough oxygen.

Answer:

true.

Asthma is relatively common during pregnancy, affecting about 7 percent of women. If treated properly, asthmatic women can have normal pregnancies. But left untreated, asthma can cause a host of problems for your baby, including growth retardation (when the baby is smaller than normal), preterm birth, and in severe cases fetal death. It can also cause problems for you too, including high blood pressure, severe nausea and vomiting, preeclampsia (a condition that can damage the mother's kidneys, brain, liver, and eyes), and labor complications.

Most asthma medications are safe for use during pregnancy. Ask your doctor about scheduling monthly lung checkups as well as periodic checks that your baby is getting enough oxygen. After 28 weeks, it's also a good idea to do daily kick counts (you want 10 kicks every two hours) and periodic ultrasounds to monitor the baby's growth. Call your doctor if you have an asthma attack. She may want to monitor your baby's heart rate and your lung function to make sure your baby wasn't deprived of oxygen during the attack.

#61

If I'm stung by a bee, can it hurt the baby?

❑ a.   Only if it hurts you (since your baby can feel your pain).

❑ b.   Only if you are severely allergic to bees.

❑ c.   Only if you were stung in the belly.

❑ d.   No, bee stings won't hurt you or your baby.

Answer:

b.

Allergies don't develop until after birth, so you don't have to worry about a sting bothering your fetus. But if bee stings put you into anaphylactic shock, you're not the only one at risk. Severe anaphylaxis can cause your airways to close, which can decrease the blood and oxygen supply to your fetus.

Women with severe bee allergies should always carry proper treatment, whether or not they're pregnant. Treating anaphylaxis with an EpiPen, which delivers an immediate dose of adrenaline to the heart, is safe during pregnancy and could save your life.

Mild allergies—the sort that make a bee sting pop out like a mosquito bite—pose no danger to a growing fetus. If the reaction bothers you or causes intense itching, you can safely treat it with antihistamines, such as Benadryl.

#62

What herbs should I avoid during pregnancy?

- ❑ a. Goldenseal, pennyroyal, and St. John's wort.
- ❑ b. Ephedra, ginkgo biloba, and yohimbe.
- ❑ c. Both a and b.
- ❑ d. Herbs are harmless during pregnancy unless laced with illegal drugs.

Answer:

C.

Most doctors recommend avoiding all herbal remedies during pregnancy—not because these are bad for you, but because they don't require FDA approval. That means they don't have to undergo the same rigorous testing and evaluation as prescription drugs and over-the-counter medications.

Some natural remedies are probably fine (ginger and peppermint, for instance, are great for relieving nausea), but some are definite no-no's. According to the Natural Medicine Database, the following herbs contain elements that can be harmful to a growing fetus:

saw palmetto
goldenseal
dong quai
ephedra
yohimbe
black cohosh

blue cohosh
Roman chamomile
pennyroyal
ginkgo biloba
St. John's wort

As always, check with your doctor before taking any medicine or herbal supplement.

#63

True or False:

Drinking a daily
cup of coffee is bad
for my unborn baby.

Answer:
false.

According to the March of Dimes, women who are pregnant or trying to become pregnant can safely consume up to 200 milligrams of caffeine per day; that's about 1 to 2 cups (not jumbo, could-be-a-soup-bowl-sized mugs) of regular coffee. A 2008 study found that women who consumed more than that daily were twice as likely to miscarry as women who were caffeine-free. And caffeine is also in

Coca-Cola (*12-ounce can*): 35 milligrams

Red Bull (*8.3-ounce can*): 76 milligrams

Black tea (*8 ounces*): 40 to 120 milligrams

Starbucks Chai tea latte (*16 ounces*): 100 milligrams

Instant powdered iced tea (*1 teaspoon*): 27 milligrams

Coffee ice cream (*200 grams*): 50 to 60 milligrams

Dark chocolate (*1.45 ounces*): 31 milligrams

Milk chocolate (*1.4 ounces*): 6 milligrams

If you're thinking it's safer to drink decaf, think again: Many manufacturers decaffeinate coffee beans using methylene chloride, which in very high doses has been found to be an animal carcinogen. The FDA maintains that chemically treated decaf is safe, but you might want to choose blends decaffeinated by a Swiss-water process instead.

#64

Could household cleaning products be dangerous for my baby?

❑ a.   Bleach can be.
❑ b.   Ammonia can be.
❑ c.   Chlorine can be.
❑ d.   No, household cleaning products aren't likely to harm your baby.

d.

According to the March of Dimes, with minimal exposure, products that contain chlorine, bleach, and ammonia (all common ingredients in cleaning products) are unlikely to harm an unborn baby. Their odors, on the other hand, may make you feel a little sick, so while cleaning be sure to keep your home well ventilated.

To be safe, wear rubber gloves to minimize contact with chemicals. Or choose all-natural cleaning products, which put ingredients such as baking soda and vinegar to working getting rid of grease and grime.

Pregnant or not, never mix ammonia with chlorine or bleach. This combination can produce chlorine gas, a toxic fume that could hurt you, your baby, and anyone else within inhaling distance.

65

True or False:

The use of air freshener can be harmful for my unborn baby.

Answer:

true.

Air freshener may smell good, but it's not so good for your little one. According to a British study of 14,000 pregnant women, children whose mothers used aerosols and air fresheners daily during pregnancy had a higher incidence of diarrhea and earaches in infancy and childhood.

If that's not convincing enough, a 2007 study by the Natural Resources Defense Council concluded that many air fresheners contain phthalates, chemicals that can affect testosterone levels and lead to reproductive abnormalities, including irregular genitalia and reduced sperm production. Doctors are most concerned about exposure to phthalates during the 8th and 15th weeks of pregnancy, when the sex organs are developing.

So how to keep your home smelling fresh without contaminating the air?

- Place stink-fighting baking soda or a little vinegar with lemon juice in small dishes around the house and invest in houseplants.
- Simmer a little vinegar on the stove while cooking to alleviate the scent of stinky foods.
- Throw a slice of lemon in the garbage disposal to reduce food-scrap smells.

66

Is it safe to pump my own gas?

❑ a.   No, the fumes can be harmful to your unborn baby.

❑ b.   No, the fumes can trigger labor.

❑ c.   Sure, as long as you don't breathe while you're pumping.

❑ d.   Sure, but just don't work as a gas station attendant.

Answer:

d.

Pumping gas is fine; hanging out by the pump all day is not. Though it's true that pregnant women should avoid exposure to volatile organic compounds (VOCs), one of which is the methanol found in gasoline, the amount you're exposed to during the occasional fill-up isn't likely to harm you or your baby.

To be safe, make sure the area is well ventilated, step away from the pump while filling up to minimize exposure to fumes, and wash your hands afterward to prevent chemical residue from seeping into your skin.

67

Didn't pregnant women years ago used to drink alcohol? Why can't I?

❏ a.　　Alcohol used to be less toxic than it is now.

❏ b.　　Women used to drink only wine, which is healthier than hard liquor.

❏ c.　　Women didn't know that it can cause fetal alcohol syndrome.

❏ d.　　Drinking alcohol is fine. People today overreact.

Answer:

C.

It's true that women used to drink throughout their pregnancies. They also used to smoke, take hot baths, and do a lot of other things we now know are dangerous to an unborn child.

The fact is, when you consume alcohol, it travels through your bloodstream and crosses the placenta to your baby. Small amounts are unlikely to cause major damage, but serious drinking can interfere with fetal development, especially during the first trimester.

The biggest concern is fetal alcohol syndrome (FAS). Usually caused by heavy drinking, FAS is marked by central nervous system problems and stunted growth. FAS babies may have problems learning, remembering, hearing, and speaking. They may also have low birth weights, display flattened facial features, and remain smaller than other children in their age group.

According to the March of Dimes, there is no "safe" amount of alcohol that can be consumed during pregnancy. At least one study has found that even a single alcoholic drink per day while pregnant may cause learning disabilities in children later on. Other studies have suggested that moderate drinking during pregnancy may increase the risk of attention deficit and hyperactivity disorder.

68

I've heard that paint releases chemicals that are bad for my baby. What is the safest way to paint the nursery?

❏ a.   Wear a mask.
❏ b.   Keep the windows open.
❏ c.   Paint the room as quickly as possible.
❏ d.   Find someone else to do the job.

Answer:
d.

Painting is a physically strenuous task, whether you're pregnant or not, and if you can get someone else to tackle the job, do it. If you must do it yourself, wear gloves and keep the room well ventilated. Consider waiting until your third trimester (the first two trimesters are the most crucial in your baby's development), and don't push yourself to finish all in one day.

VOC-free formulas are the way to go. VOCs are the gases released into the air as paint dries (and what make some paints smell so strong). In the short term, these gases can cause headaches and dizziness. Long-term effects are less certain, but some studies have linked frequent VOC exposure to miscarriages and birth defects.

After VOC-free formulas, water- or latex-based paints are the next best choice. Lead-based paints are no longer sold; if your house was built before 1970, however, lead paint may already be on the walls. Have someone else scrape off and sand the old paint. Stay out of the house while the work's being done since inhaling lead dust could be harmful to you and your baby.

#69

True or False:

Traveling by plane during pregnancy can harm my baby.

Answer:
false.

The safest time to fly is in the second trimester, according to the American College of Obstetricians and Gynecologists, but only because it's after the period when most miscarriages naturally occur and before you're at risk for early labor. (Either scenario will be more difficult if it occurs while you're in the air; the flight itself won't cause them.) After about 35 weeks, flying is not recommended, since 30,000 feet in the air isn't exactly the safest place for labor and delivery.

To stay comfortable during the flight, try to:

- Book an aisle seat. Most pregnant women go to the bathroom about once an hour, and sitting on the aisle makes these frequent visits less disruptive.
- Avoid gassy foods and carbonated drinks. Gas expands in the cabin's low air pressure and may cause uncomfortable (though not unsafe) bloating.
- Wear your seatbelt. You'll be happy you did when turbulence hits.
- Stretch your legs. Get up and walk around every few hours to avoid deep vein thrombosis, a condition common among air travelers in which dangerous blood clots form in the legs. Wearing support panty hose can also help.

70

If I'm afraid of flying, what can I take to relax during a flight?

- ❏ a.　Certain anti-anxiety medications.
- ❏ b.　A glass of wine.
- ❏ c.　Benadryl.
- ❏ d.　All of the above.

Answer:

d.

Some anti-anxiety medications can be taken during pregnancy (ask your doctor), but none are considered 100 percent safe. That said, severe stress and anxiety aren't good for your baby, either, so discuss with your doctor whether improving your mental health is worth the risks of taking medication.

Many women find that a single dose of Benadryl is strong enough to make them feel drowsy and relaxed. For some, a one-time glass of wine helps to ease stress and shouldn't hurt the baby either.

Of course, you can always try natural stress-reduction techniques. Now might be the time to experiment with such age-old methods as deep breathing and meditation. If you need extra help, stock up on books and CDs specifically about tackling the fear of flying.

#71

What happens if I go into labor on a plane?

❏ a.   The plane must turn around to get you to your own hospital.

❏ b.   You have to pay for the plane to land at the nearest airport.

❏ c.   Flight attendants and other passengers would help you deliver your baby if the plane couldn't land in time.

❏ d.   The air pressure would likely delay your labor to give you time to get to a hospital at your destination.

Answer:

C.

Going into labor at 30,000 feet certainly isn't ideal, but if that's when your baby is ready to come out, there's nothing you can do. If you feel contractions while in the air, speak up. The flight crew must divert the plane to get you to a hospital; they'll also make sure there's an ambulance waiting as soon as you land.

Of course, there's always the chance you'll land with your baby in your arms rather than in your belly. With 200-plus passengers, chances are good that a doctor or nurse would be on board to help with the delivery. If not, flight attendants may be able to do the job.

Yet even though flight crews are trained to deal with unexpected deliveries, most airlines try to avoid such emergencies by barring pregnant women close to their due dates from flying at all. Each airline has a different policy: some don't let women fly after 36 weeks; others let pregnant women fly until their due date, provided they have a doctor's note.

72

Can I wear a bikini while sporting a "baby bump"?

❑ a.   No, sun on your belly can increase your baby's chance of getting cancer later in life.

❑ b.   No, sun on your belly can heat up the temperature of your uterus, which can be dangerous to your baby.

❑ c.   Sure, but wear a good sunblock since your skin is more sun-sensitive during pregnancy.

❑ d.   Sure, a little sun is good for you both.

Answer:

C.

Sunbathing won't hurt your baby (your skin may feel hot, but it won't change the temperature in your womb), but it's certainly not good for your skin.

Pregnancy hormones make your skin extra sensitive, which means that a 30-minute sunbathing session that used to tan you perfectly might now cause a killer sunburn. That may put you at increased risk for skin cancer later in life. If that's not enough, tanning during pregnancy may also contribute to the darkening of your skin, known as the "mask of pregnancy," which can cause permanent dark spots on your face and belly.

Stay in the shade. If you must be exposed, avoid peak hours (10 am to 2 pm), wear a hat, and use a broad-spectrum sunblock with an SPF of at least 30.

#73

Is it safe to go boating?

❏ a. Only in the first trimester, when the bumps
         in the water won't bother your baby.

❏ b. Only if the water isn't too rough.

❏ c. Only if you're an experienced boater.

❏ d. Only if you're having a boy.

Answer:

b.

Boating is safe as long as you're not sailing rough seas. A leisurely paddle is fine; white-water rafting on class-four rapids probably isn't.

In general, avoid situations in which you could be tossed around. Most bumps aren't strong enough to bother your baby (who's safely cushioned inside your uterus), but rough waters may cause you to fall or something to fall into you. Also, since morning sickness may be exacerbated by motion, you might want to wait until your second trimester to hit the water. Pregnancy may worsen motion sickness, so if you usually get queasy on boats, you're better off embracing your landlubber side.

Either way, stay close to shore, especially as you near your due date. The last place you want to go into labor is in the middle of the ocean.

74

At what point in my pregnancy should I ask my partner to stop taking business trips?

☐ a.   At 32 weeks.
☐ b.   At 34 weeks.
☐ c.   At 37 weeks.
☐ d.   It depends where he's going.

Answer:

d.

Faraway destinations are risky, since your partner may not be back in time once your labor begins. Yet even if he's out of town when you feel your first contraction, chances are he'll be able to get home before your baby is born. Most first-time moms have 12 to 24 hours (or more) between their first contraction and delivery. Subsequent births take about half as long. Still, about 12 percent of babies in the United States are born prematurely. You may be at risk if

- You've had a previous preterm delivery.
- You're pregnant with multiples.
- You're younger than 17 or older than 35.
- You're African American (according to the March of Dimes, African American women are most likely to give birth at least three weeks early).
- You didn't gain enough weight during pregnancy.
- You were underweight before you got pregnant.
- You have a shortened cervix.
- You are shorter than 5 feet.
- You smoked, abused alcohol, or used drugs during pregnancy.
- You became pregnant within six months of giving birth to your previous child.

75

Why is it dangerous to visit volcanoes?

❏ a.   If the volcano erupts, you may not be able to run fast enough to get out of harm's way.

❏ b.   Your balance is off during pregnancy, so you risk falling into the volcano.

❏ c.   Volcanic fumes may be toxic to your unborn baby.

❏ d.   Volcanic ash can land on your skin and enter your bloodstream.

Answer:

C.

Volcanic fumes contain toxins that may be harmful to pregnant women as well as young children, infants, and people with known respiratory conditions such as asthma.

They are a common concern in Hawaii, where residents have suffered a wide range of health problems due to what they call "vog" (volcanic fog), the visible haze produced when sulfur dioxide and other volcanic gases combine with chemicals in the atmosphere. Vog has been found to contain small amounts of several toxic metals, including selenium, mercury, arsenic, and iridium. Health effects from exposure include headaches, breathing difficulties, and flulike symptoms.

It's unclear what effect these fumes have on an unborn baby, but the danger is severe enough that the National Park Service discourages pregnant women from visiting volcanic parks altogether.

Seeing the park from your car may not be safer. Fumes can linger in the air for several miles, so if you're in your car and see a haze, close the windows and turn the air conditioning to the recycled-air setting. Also, keep your radio tuned to National Park Service advisories on air quality in the area.

76

True or False:

You shouldn't use the shoulder-strap portion of a seat belt during pregnancy.

Answer:

false.

Not only is it safe to wear a seat belt the correct way, it could save your life. (Plus, it's required by law in the United States). According to a study published in the *American Journal of Obstetrics and Gynecology*, almost 200 fetuses a year—or half of all fetal losses due to motor vehicle crashes—could be saved if pregnant women had buckled up correctly.

Though there is a slight risk of an air bag deploying force-fully enough to cause injury or complications, the American College of Obstetricians and Gynecologists still advises preg-nant women not to deactivate their air bags since the benefits outweigh possible dangers. To minimize the risk of air-bag injuries, experts suggest sitting as far back as possible (at least 10 inches) from the dashboard or steering wheel.

Buckle that bump! Here's how to buckle up your belly:

- Make sure the lap portion of the belt sits below your abdomen, as low on your hips as possible.
- Never place the belt above or atop your belly.
- Adjust the shoulder strap so that it lies between the breasts, below the neck.

77

True or False:

Being at high altitudes can affect your pregnancy.

Answer:
true.

Whether or not you can travel to high-altitude destinations depends on how high you want to go. A trip to Vail, Colorado, isn't going to cause any problems; climbing Mount Kilimanjaro, on the other hand, isn't a good idea.

The Centers for Disease Control and Prevention advises pregnant women to avoid altitudes above 12,000 feet. That's because the higher you go, the less oxygen there is, which makes breathing difficult. And less oxygen for you means less oxygen for your baby. In fact, studies have found that women living at high altitudes are more likely to give birth to smaller babies.

But it's not just the altitude you should worry about. High-altitude destinations are often found in remote locations, far from the medical care you'd need should an emergency arise.

If you're spending time in higher elevations during your pregnancy, be sure to take things slowly. With less oxygen in the air, you'll get tired a lot more quickly than usual. Take frequent breaks and, if you feel dizzy or lightheaded, sit down and rest.

#78

What harm can jogging exert on my baby?

❏ a.   It could cause miscarriages.

❏ b.   It could jostle your baby, which could affect brain development.

❏ c.   It won't hurt your baby, but you may want to cut back once your belly gets too big.

❏ d.   It won't hurt your baby, but it may turn him around in the womb.

Answer:

C.

Exercise can help stave off excess baby weight, and it's been shown to alleviate labor pains and help women more quickly recover from childbirth. As long as you're having a healthy pregnancy, jogging won't bother your baby, but it may be hard on you. Thanks to the hormone relaxin working to soften your joints and ligaments (it's what helps loosen your pelvis to push out the baby), any exercise during pregnancy puts you at greater risk for muscle sprains, strains, and tears. Jogging on a treadmill instead of the open road will be easier on your joints.

No matter your activity, stay hydrated, avoid overheating, and always stop exercising if you feel dizzy or faint. If you have any of the following conditions, ask your doctor if exercise is advisable:

- a heart condition
- restrictive lung disease or asthma
- an incompetent cervix
- a risk for premature labor
- persistent bleeding
- placenta previa
- ruptured membranes
- pregnancy-induced hypertension
- poorly controlled diabetes

#79

What yoga poses should I avoid?

❑ a.   Any in which you're lying on your back.
❑ b.   Any in which you put weight on your abdomen.
❑ c.   Bikram (aka "hot") yoga.
❑ d.   All of the above.

Answer:

d.

Yoga can be a great way to stay fit and relaxed while you're expecting. Besides increasing flexibility and strength, deep breathing and meditation used by certain yoga practices can decrease stress and anxiety during pregnancy, labor, and delivery. Tell the instructor you're pregnant so she can modify (or eliminate) poses that may be unsafe. Or consider taking a prenatal yoga class.

Although no studies have examined the consequences of practicing yoga during pregnancy, you should avoid poses that put weight on your abdomen, including bow, cobra, locust, plow, peacock, crane, shoulderstand, and headstand. Beginning around 20 weeks, avoid lying flat on your back, since this can affect blood flow and nutrient supply to the uterus. A few minutes in corpse pose probably won't hurt, but it may constrict blood flow just enough to leave you lightheaded.

Remember that your joints and tissues have softened, so although it may feel like you can pretzel yourself into a plethora of new positions, you might overdo it. And don't do Bikram, or "hot," yoga. Working out in hot temperatures may leave you overheated, which could harm the fetus.

80

Can I do sit-ups?

❏ a.   No, it might strain the muscles of your uterus.
❏ b.   No, it's not good to lie on your back.
❏ c.   Sure, sit-ups are fine during pregnancy.
❏ d.   Sure, but only if you were overweight before pregnancy.

Answer:

b.

During pregnancy, you may want to avoid the traditional sit-up, which is done while lying flat on the back. Particularly in the second and third trimesters, lying on your back can put weight on the major veins that bring blood back to the heart. If they are obstructed for an extended period, the flow of nutrients to your baby may be affected. In the short term, it can make you feel lightheaded and dizzy.

Still, strengthening your core muscles can help alleviate pregnancy-related back pain and the poor posture caused by a bulging belly. Experts say it may also help with labor and delivery. Instead of sit-ups, try pelvic tilt exercises, which are safe to do during pregnancy. To do them:

1. Get down on all fours with your arms shoulder-width apart and your knees hip-width apart. Keep your arms straight without locking your elbows.
2. As you breathe in, tighten your abdominal muscles, tuck your butt in toward your belly, and round your back.
3. Relax your back into a neutral position as you breathe out.
4. Repeat. Aim for three sets of 10 at least once a day.

81

Can I continue my rock-climbing activities?

❏ a.   Only during your first trimester.
❏ b.   Only if you were climbing before you
          became pregnant.
❏ c.   Only if your belly can fit into the harness.
❏ d.   No, rock climbing is too risky during
          pregnancy.

Answer:

a.

Rock climbing shouldn't be a problem in your first trimester, especially if you're an experienced climber. After that, it's not recommended because your uterus will have grown beyond the protective shell of your pelvis and your baby will be more vulnerable to injury should you lose your grip and collide with a rock. Keep in mind, too, that you're more prone to sprains and other injuries, thanks to the hormone relaxin.

To be safe, during pregnancy many climbers switch to bouldering. Bouldering doesn't require ropes, and climbers are never more than a few feet off the ground. Falling is less of an issue, since climbers move sideways instead of upward.

If you're going to climb, make sure you do so on routes you know. Now's not the time to experiment with a new rock face. A better choice is an indoor climbing gym, which has padded floors and plenty of help should you need it. And always wear a harness, specifically one designed to be worn below the belly to avoid putting undue pressure on your abdomen.

82

True or False:

The chemicals in chlorinated pools can be harmful to an unborn baby.

Answer:
false.

As long as you're not ingesting large amounts of pool water, the chlorine won't hurt you or your baby. In fact, chlorine has an important job to do: It kills germs almost instantly, which is a definite advantage when you consider all the icky things that could be lurking in a pool. Plus, swimming is an excellent low-impact activity and a great way to stay cool during pregnancy.

However, swimming in an unchlorinated pool or a pond is risky. The water could be teeming with bacteria and viruses, including salmonella, E. coli, hepatitis A, staphylococcus, and giardia. A pregnant woman is more vulnerable to infections from these pathogens, since her immune system is naturally suppressed. Some of these organisms can also cross the placenta and infect the fetus, which can result in miscarriage, stillbirth, premature labor, or other complications.

83

Is horseback riding safe?

❑ a.   Yes, as long as you're an experienced rider and you stop by your second trimester.
❑ b.   Yes, as long as you know the horse well.
❑ c.   No, it's never safe to ride during pregnancy because the risk of falling or being kicked by the horse is too great.
❑ d.   No, because horses are skittish around pregnant women.

Answer:

a.

If you're an experienced equestrian, it may be fine to continue riding during the first trimester. After that, your baby bump might shift your center of gravity and render you off-balance, and your bodily changes may make sitting astride a horse uncomfortable.

The real danger, pregnant or not, is falling. (Indeed, according to a six-year analysis of sports in England and Wales, riding was found to be more hazardous than air sports, motor sports, or mountaineering.) Riding at a fast pace or on hilly or rocky terrain is discouraged, no matter how saddle-savvy you are. Falling off a horse could injure the fetus or cause a miscarriage, especially during your second or third trimester when the fetus is no longer protected by your pelvic bones. If you are at risk for preterm labor, you may want to refrain from riding altogether, since the jarring bumps of your horse's gait could put enough pressure on your cervix to induce labor. If you have partial or complete placenta previa (when the placenta covers the cervix), riding can also cause bleeding or other complications.

84

Can I still do my favorite dances?

❏ a.   Ballroom dancing is fine; hip-hop and ballet are too strenuous.

❏ b.   Dancing is fine as long as you're not a professional dancer.

❏ c.   After your first trimester, dance away.

❏ d.   As long as your pregnancy is healthy, cut a rug as often as you like.

Answer:

d.

Most styles of dance are fine during pregnancy. As long as you're healthy, the general rule of thumb is this: If you were doing it before you got pregnant, you can continue it throughout your pregnancy.

However, you'll soon find that dancing for two is a little more challenging. For one, you'll probably get tired faster. When you're pregnant, your heart pumps 30 to 50 percent more blood through your body—and exercising makes it work even harder. That shouldn't be dangerous for you or your baby, but it'll poop you out pretty quickly. Staying hydrated and stopping when you're tired are also important, since overheating and overexertion aren't good for you or your baby. To prevent muscle sprains, strains, and tears, avoid moves that require sudden turns, and keep at least one foot on the ground at all times.

Women at risk for preterm labor may want to stay off the dance floor—or stick to slow dancing—throughout their pregnancies. In addition, talk to your doctor before embarking on any exercise program, especially if you have a heart or lung condition, poorly controlled diabetes, an incompetent cervix, persistent bleeding, ruptured membranes, or placenta previa.

85

Can I jump on a trampoline?

❑ a.   Yes, as long as you have a safety net.
❑ b.   Yes, as long as you don't do any flips.
❑ c.   Yes, but only in your second trimester.
❑ d.   No, jumping on a trampoline is never safe.

Answer:
d.

Trampolines are not safe, whether you're pregnant or not. According to the U.S. Consumer Product Safety Commission (CPSC), emergency rooms treat more than 80,000 trampoline-related injuries per year—making them more dangerous than skateboards, bikes, or rollerblades.

The biggest danger is that you'll lose your balance and fall, which becomes ever more likely as your belly gets bigger and your center of gravity shifts to accommodate your baby bump. Another concern is that the pounding pressure of your uterus on your cervix could cause contractions that may potentially trigger preterm labor. That's an even bigger worry if you're already at risk for an early delivery or if you've had changes in your cervix. You should also worry about minor injuries. Trampolining isn't easy on the body, and an errant landing may seriously strain your joints. Your bladder won't like it either. Urinary incontinence is common during pregnancy, and jumping will only worsen the problem.

86

Pregnant cross-country skiing—safe or not?

❏ a.   Yes, as long as you stick to flat terrain.
❏ b.   Yes, as long as you don't go above 12,000 feet.
❏ c.   Yes, as long as you're an experienced skier.
❏ d.   All of the above.

Answer:
d.

Cross-country skiing while pregnant is OK as long as you know what you're doing. If you're not experienced, now's not the time to take up the sport.

Though there have been no reports of birth defects resulting from high-altitude exposure during pregnancy, the Centers for Disease Control and Prevention recommends that pregnant women stay below 12,000 feet to avoid any possible complications. At the least, the reduced oxygen in the air may make you dizzy or lightheaded. High altitudes can also tire you out a lot more quickly, so be sure to stop when you feel fatigued.

If you're in your third trimester—and especially if you're at risk for early labor—be careful to stay close to civilization. You don't want to be stuck on the slopes when you feel your first contraction.

Under no circumstances should you engage in downhill skiing while pregnant, since there's always a risk of falling. A spill can be especially hazardous after the first trimester, when the baby is no longer protected by your pelvic bones.

87

True or False:

Pregnant women shouldn't jump rope.

Answer:
false.

The impact on your cervix while jumping rope isn't that different from jogging at a moderate pace. As long as you haven't had problems or changes in your cervix (have your doctor check), this activity shouldn't cause problems for you or your baby.

But if your cervix is shortened or dilated, or if you've been told that you're at risk for premature labor, you might want to find another form of exercise. The repetitive pounding of your uterus on your cervix may be enough pressure to trigger contractions and, ultimately, early labor. Yoga or swimming may be a better choice.

Stop jumping immediately if you feel contractions. Most likely, they're just Braxton-Hicks contractions—harmless "practice" contractions that tend to worsen after exercise. These usually last no longer than 15 to 20 minutes; however, if they don't go away or if they're coming at regular intervals, call your doctor.

88

Can I skydive?

- ❏ a.   Yes, but only if you use a special kind of parachute.
- ❏ b.   Yes, but only if you wear an oxygen mask.
- ❏ c.   Yes, but only in the second trimester.
- ❏ d.   It's been done—but it's not a good idea.

Answer:

d.

Contrary to what you might think, it isn't the 124-mile-per-hour plummet that poses a danger to your unborn baby; it's the pull of your parachute. This sudden slowdown can exert enough force to sheer the placenta away from the wall of the uterus (similar to the effects of a car accident). This condition, called placental abruption, is a life-threatening situation for both mother and baby.

Even if the dive doesn't hurt your baby, it might hurt you. You're now more vulnerable to sprains and strains, thanks to the extra hormones working to loosen your joints (to ultimately help you push during labor). And, of course, there's a chance of landing belly-first. Or landing on an electrical wire. Or a highway. Why take such risks when you're a mommy-to-be?

That said, it has been done. In 2005, 21-year-old Shayna Richardson landed face-first on the asphalt after her parachute failed to open properly. She didn't know she was pregnant, and both she and her baby survived. For the sake of your baby: Stay grounded.

89

Is it all right to attend a loud rock concert?

❑ a.   Sure, just don't body surf.
❑ b.   Sure, you should have fun while you can.
❑ c.   No, the music may be too loud for your baby.
❑ d.   No, the crowds may be too raucous.

Answer:

a.

As long as you're not being overly jostled and bumped in the belly, the occasional rock concert poses no threat to you or your baby.

That said, you may not want to stand next to the speakers. By week 30, your baby's eardrums are fully developed, meaning that he hears almost everything you hear. Most of it is muffled, but research has found that low-pitch sounds, such as a bass guitar, are amplified by amniotic fluid.

One-time exposure to loud noise isn't likely to hurt your baby, but it may not be good for you. Research has shown that even one minute of noise above 110 decibels could cause permanent hearing damage, whether or not you're pregnant. (Pregnant women who spend eight hours a day around loud noise may give birth to babies with hearing problems.)

One last word of caution: Should you blast an eardrum, you'll have to brave it out. Treatment for a blown eardrum (namely, heavy-duty pain meds) is contraindicated during pregnancy.

90

True or False:

Gardening can
be dangerous for
pregnant women.

Answer:

true.

There's no need to stop tending your plants and vegetables during these nine months, but you'll want to take precautions. Keep clear of chemical pesticides, which contain toxins known to cause birth defects and miscarriages after repeated or long-term exposure. Always read the warnings on your plant and flower sprays; even so-called natural pesticides can be harmful.

Working in the garden may put you at risk for toxoplasmosis, an infection caused by a parasite found in contaminated animal (usually cat) feces. You come into contact with it when you dig up dirt where an infected animal has defecated. Toxoplasmosis could cause serious problems for your baby, including mental retardation, brain damage, or even death. Many people, especially cat owners, are already immune to toxoplasmosis; ask your doctor to test you. If you had the infection before pregnancy, you can't get it again or pass it on to your baby. To keep smelling (and planting) the roses, remember to:

- Wear rubber gloves.
- Wash your hands thoroughly after gardening.
- Thoroughly wash all produce before consuming.
- Don't lift heavy bags of soil or other large, weighty objects.

91

Is scuba diving safe?

❑ a.   No, it can be dangerous because your baby can't properly decompress.

❑ b.   No, it can be dangerous because your belly can make you sink too deep.

❑ c.   Yes, but only if you're an expert diver.

❑ d.   Yes, but only during the first trimester.

Answer:

a.

Studies have shown a higher risk of birth defects and preterm
birth among women who scuba dive during pregnancy. The
deeper you dive, the higher the risk.

The biggest danger is decompression sickness, commonly
known as "the bends," which sets in when a diver swims to the
surface too quickly and the sudden change in pressure releases
trapped nitrogen gases in the body. It's a potentially fatal
condition usually avoided by divers carefully decompressing
during their ascent. A growing baby, however, cannot properly
decompress, so there is a risk that scuba diving may leave dangerous trapped gas bubbles in the baby's circulatory system.
In addition, if the mother were to get decompression sickness,
it could be harmful for the fetus. To further complicate things,
the common treatment for the condition—recompressing in a
hyperbaric oxygen chamber—could also pose risks to the baby.

Save scuba till after your baby is born. For now, try snor-
keling, which is safe during pregnancy. Just avoid ponds or
fresh-water lagoons, which are more likely to harbor harmful
bacteria.

92

True or False:

Unborn babies can taste the foods their mothers eat.

Answer:

true.

Studies suggest that once your baby is at least 28 weeks in the womb, he may be able to taste what you're eating. Taste buds develop around 9 weeks after conception, though the brain connections that help distinguish tastes aren't fully functional until near the beginning of the third trimester. By this time, your baby is swallowing amniotic fluid by the mouthful and is likely tasting hints of flavors from your meals, especially if you're eating potent spices such as garlic and curry powder, which have been shown to be strong enough to change the odor of amniotic fluid.

What you're eating while you're expecting may also influence your baby's taste preferences after birth, according to a study at Philadelphia's Monell Chemical Senses Center. Researchers assigned 46 pregnant women to one of three groups: Those in one drank carrot juice daily; the second group drank water and then carrot juice daily; and the third avoided carrot juice altogether. After the babies began eating solid foods, researchers offered them a choice of plain cereal or cereal mixed with carrot juice. Babies whose mothers drank carrot juice while pregnant ate more carrot-flavored cereal and showed fewer negative facial responses to it than babies whose moms had avoided carrot juice.

93

What's the problem with using a microwave oven?

❏ a.   Eating microwaved food increases the chances your baby will later develop cancer.

❏ b.   Microwaved food has fewer nutrients.

❏ c.   Microwave ovens emit radiation, which can cause problems in unborn babies.

❏ d.   There's no problem . . . as long as you're not using an antiquated microwave.

Answer:
d.

All microwaves made after 1971 are shielded to reduce microwave radiation levels to extremely low levels (and even before
1971, it's unlikely that leaky microwaves caused health problems). Nowadays, you'd have to be sitting inside the microwave
for it to cause any damage to you or your baby.

Contrary to public opinion, standing near a microwave or
eating microwaved food poses no proven risks. You may call it
"nuking" food, but in reality microwave radiation (which is not
the same as nuclear radiation) is in the same electromagnetic
class as radio waves and is, therefore, harmless.

Regulations imposed by the U.S. Food and Drug
Administration limit the amount of microwaves that can leak
from an oven, which is why the ovens won't work with an
open door. Microwave radiation dissipates the farther you are
from the source, so if you're still worried about the potential
effects of exposure, standing even a few feet away will keep
you safe.

And, if you're still using a pre-1971 microwave oven, sell it
to an antiques store.

94

True or False:

Feta cheese is safe to
eat during pregnancy.

Answer:
false.

Feta is one cheese that should be avoided during pregnancy. That's because it—along with other unpasteurized cheeses such as Brie, Camembert, and goat's milk—may be contaminated with listeria, a bacteria that makes adults sick and can be dangerous for unborn babies. Symptoms of listeriosis occur 2 to 30 days after exposure to the bacteria and include flulike symptoms, headaches, nausea, and vomiting. If you notice any of these after having eaten feta cheese, see your doctor, who will prescribe antibiotics to fight the infection before it can affect your baby.

Of course, most cheeses, unpasteurized or not, are contaminant-free, so if you've eaten only a little bit, chances are you'll be fine. Just avoid it from here on out. In the future, stick with hard or semisoft cheeses such as cheddar and mozzarella. Pasteurized cheese slices and spreads such as cream cheese and cottage cheese are also OK. (In addition, some feta and Brie varieties are pasteurized; check the labels.) Also, cooking kills bacteria, so fully cooked cheese is fine to eat.

95

What's wrong with eating peanut butter?

- ❏ a.   It makes your baby more likely to develop a nut allergy.
- ❏ b.   Your baby might have an allergic reaction in the womb.
- ❏ c.   Your baby will be born hating peanuts.
- ❏ d.   Probably nothing.

Answer:

d.

Peanuts are a good source of protein, unsaturated fat, fiber, niacin, calcium, and minerals. They make a great snack for the nutrient-needy pregnant woman.

But are they safe? The jury is still out. Some studies have suggested that eating peanut butter while pregnant increases a baby's likelihood of developing a peanut allergy; other studies have shown no link between the two. Until recently, the American Academy of Pediatrics advised pregnant women to avoid peanuts; however, in 2008 they reversed their position, saying that no evidence indicates that restrictions in a mother's diet reduce the likelihood of allergies.

If your family has a history of nut allergies—especially if one of your children has a food allergy—some doctors recommend limiting your consumption of nuts while you're pregnant and breastfeeding, which will give your baby's immune system a chance to fully mature. You should also wait until your child is 3 years old before introducing peanuts into his diet.

If you do choose to limit your nut intake, alternatives such as soy nut butter, sunflower seed butter, and hemp butter may satisfy your cravings.

96

Which of the following foods are safe to eat during pregnancy?

❏ a.   Homemade mayonnaise, eggnog, and Caesar dressing.
❏ b.   Scrambled eggs, hard-boiled eggs, and omelets.
❏ c.   Cake batter and raw cookie dough.
❏ d.   Mousse and meringue.

Answer:

b.

Uncooked eggs may be teeming with salmonella, a potentially dangerous bacteria. Because pregnant women have weakened immune systems, they are particularly vulnerable to salmonella infection. Symptoms develop within 12 to 72 hours of ingestion and include fever, stomach cramps, nausea, vomiting, and diarrhea. If you think you might be infected, contact your doctor immediately. Though the infection doesn't usually affect the baby, the dehydration caused by diarrhea and vomiting could cause a miscarriage. Rarely, salmonella infection can cross the placenta and cause serious complications including preterm birth, severe illness, miscarriage, or fetal death.

To prevent exposure, cook eggs fully—that is, until the whites are white and the yolks are solid—and don't eat foods containing raw eggs, especially homemade mayonnaise or eggnog, raw cake or cookie batter, mousse, and meringue.

When dining out, ask the restaurant manager if the dressings contain raw eggs. Store-bought products made with pasteurized eggs are safe to eat. At home, don't use eggs after their "best before" date or if the shells are broken. After handling eggs, remember to wash your hands, utensils, and nearby surfaces.

97

Is it OK if I give up eating meat during pregnancy?

❏ a.   No, meat contains nutrients that can't be found in a vegetarian diet.

❏ b.   No, meat contains hormones that help your baby grow.

❏ c.   Yes, but only after the first trimester.

❏ d.   Yes, but you may need a supplement.

Answer:
d.

Remember to eat enough protein, especially iron, vitamin B12, and vitamin D, all of which are hard to obtain from vegetarian sources. According to the American College of Obstetricians and Gynecologists, pregnant women should have at least 5 to 5½ ounces of meat or beans a day, plus at least 6 ounces of grains, 2½ cups of vegetables, 2 cups of fruit, and either 3 cups of milk or 3 ounces of cheese. Here's what you need:

- **Calcium.** How much: 1,000 milligrams a day. Meatless sources: milk, cheese, yogurt.
- **Iron.** How much: 27 milligrams a day. Meatless sources: dried beans and peas, iron-fortified cereals, prune juice.
- **Vitamin A.** How much: 770 micrograms a day. Meatless sources: carrots, dark leafy greens, sweet potatoes.
- **Vitamin C.** How much: 85 milligrams a day. Meatless sources: citrus fruits, broccoli, tomatoes, strawberries.
- **Vitamin B6.** How much: 1.9 milligrams a day. Meatless sources: whole-grain cereals, bananas.
- **Vitamin B12.** How much: 2.6 micrograms a day. Meatless sources: milk (vegans must take a supplement).
- **Folate.** How much: 600 micrograms a day. Meatless sources: leafy vegetables, orange juice, legumes, nuts.

[#]**98**

What's wrong with eating a lot of sweets?

❏ a.   Too much sugar can cause cavities, which
         you're more prone to get during pregnancy.
❏ b.   Too much sugar can cause excess weight
         gain—for both you and your baby.
❏ c.   Too much sugar can make you less likely to
         eat healthy foods.
❏ d.   All of the above.

Answer:

d.

Sugar is a common pregnancy craving. In fact, some scientists believe that a pregnant woman's sweet tooth has an evolutionary basis: In our hunter-gatherer days, sweeter-tasting vegetation was higher in nutrients, whereas bitter plants were more likely to be toxic.

Indulging too much can lead to weight gain and put you at risk for high blood pressure and early delivery. Filling up on sugar may also mean you're missing the nutritious foods you need for a healthy pregnancy, and it's especially bad for your teeth, since increased progesterone levels during pregnancy make you more susceptible to tooth decay and gum disease. Both conditions have been linked to preterm labor.

Your kiddo faces plenty of problems, too. A 2007 study of 23,000 pregnant women in nine countries found a link between a mother's blood sugar levels and her chances of delivering a big baby. Large babies are at risk for shoulder damage if delivered vaginally, and they're more likely to have low blood-sugar levels and high insulin levels, problems that can later lead to obesity, diabetes, and high blood pressure.

99

Which of the following sushi restaurant items is safe to eat?

- ❏ a.   California roll.
- ❏ b.   Spicy tuna roll.
- ❏ c.   Mackerel sashimi.
- ❏ d.   None of the above.

Answer:

a.

Every time you eat raw food—whether sushi or an extrarare hamburger—you take the chance that your food is contaminated with bacteria, viruses, or parasites that could make you sick. When you're pregnant, whatever's lurking in your food poses a particular danger, since your immune system is naturally suppressed and therefore less equipped to fight infection. Food poisoning may not hurt your baby, but dehydration caused by excessive vomiting or diarrhea could cause contractions and send you into early labor. There's also a small chance that the infection may cross the placenta and infect your baby, which could cause serious consequences such as preterm birth, miscarriage, or severe illness in the newborn.

Symptoms of food-borne illnesses usually become apparent within 24 hours, so if you accidentally ate some sushi before learning of the danger and survived the dining experience without a subsequent bout of diarrhea and vomiting, you're probably fine.

From here on out, stick to the cooked stuff (California rolls, tempura rolls) and vegetable rolls. Ask the sushi chef to cut your rolls using a new knife and cutting board to minimize the risk of cross-contamination.

100

Is it worth the extra money to eat organic foods?

❏ a.   Only during the first trimester, when your
         baby is more vulnerable to toxic chemicals.
❏ b.   Only when it comes to thin-skinned pro-
         duce like peaches and apples.
❏ c.   Only if you have a lot of money.
❏ d.   Save your money—conventional foods
         are fine.

Answer:

b.

Studies haven't found adverse health effects from consuming the low levels of pesticides found in most U.S. foods; however, these chemicals can cross the placenta. So if you want to make sure your baby is toxin-free, be careful what you eat.

Fruits and vegetables tend to absorb the highest load of pesticides. Fruits with thick skins, such as papayas and mangoes, aren't as worrisome as those with thin skins, which include peaches, apples, bell peppers, celery, nectarines, strawberries, cherries, pears, imported grapes, spinach, lettuce, and potatoes.

According to the U.S. Department of Agriculture, crops certified as organic must be grown without synthetic pesticides, artificial fertilizers, or irradiation (a form of radiation used to kill bacteria). Animals from organic farms must eat organically grown feed (as opposed to feed made from animal parts), be allowed exercise or access to the outdoors, and be raised without antibiotics or growth hormones.

Of course, even organic fruits and veggies may be contaminated with bacteria or viruses. So wash all produce thoroughly before eating. Peeling helps, too, though it can also remove valuable nutrients.

101

True or False:

Twins can accidentally hurt each other in the womb.

Answer:
false.

Your twins won't hurt each other—at least not until they're toddlers. In the womb, each fetus has its own amniotic sac that acts as a buffer against in-utero antics. However, research indicates that twins and other multiples do interact with each other in the womb. Ultrasound videos have shown babies pushing, kicking, and even what looks like playing and kissing each other.

Rarely—in about 1 in 45,000 pregnancies—do identical twins share a single amniotic sac. (Your doctor will know since it's apparent on ultrasound scans.) In these cases, there is a danger that the umbilical cords will become entangled or compressed as the babies move around each other. Compression and entanglement can cut off the flow of nutrients and oxygen, so mothers are closely monitored throughout their pregnancies. As an added precaution, their babies are usually delivered early via C-section.

102

It's possible for twins to have different fathers if...

❏ a.   The mother releases two eggs in one cycle.
❏ b.   The mother has sex with two men around the same time.
❏ c.   Both of the above.
❏ d.   None of the above. Twins always have the same father.

Answer:

C.

Superfecundation, the condition in which fraternal twins have different fathers, occurs when a woman releases two eggs in one cycle. Normally, the result is fraternal twins with one dad. But if the woman engages in sex with two men around the same time, sperm can commingle in the fight to fertilize. The result: two babies, two dads. Studies suggests it happens in up to 2 percent of fraternal twin births, but it generally goes unnoticed since most parents don't consider doing a paternity test on twins.

#103

Can one twin steal food from the other in utero?

- ❏ a. Only if he's really hungry.
- ❏ b. Only if the placenta isn't working properly.
- ❏ c. Only if the mother isn't eating enough.
- ❏ d. Only if one of the babies is sick and needs more food than the other.

Answer:

b.

Twins can't technically steal food since they get their nourishment through individual umbilical cords. In cases where babies share a placenta (about half the time with identical twins), the placenta usually distributes blood flow evenly so that both babies get the right amount of oxygen and nutrients. But about 10 percent of identical twins suffer from twin–twin transfusion syndrome (TTTS). For these twins, placental blood connections are abnormal, and blood is distributed unevenly to the two fetuses. The result: One gets too much blood flow; the other too little. Severe cases can be fatal for both fetuses.

Your doctor can diagnose TTTS on an ultrasound. Telltale signs include

- a marked size difference in fetuses of the same sex
- a difference in amniotic sac or umbilical cord size
- a single placenta
- excess or decreased amniotic fluid for one of the babies

Doctors can treat the condition by performing an amniocentesis to drain excess fluid and improve blood flow. Also, laser surgery can seal the connection between the blood vessels. Both techniques save about 60 percent of affected twins.

104

True or False:

It's possible for an ultrasound not to detect a twin.

Answer:
true.

Although unlikely, it is possible for a doctor not to spot both twins if an ultrasound is performed only in the early weeks of pregnancy. But by the time kicking begins, usually between 20 and 24 weeks, it's rare for that extra pair of feet to go unnoticed.

There are cases of women who didn't know they were having twins until their second baby came down the birth canal, but that usually occurs when women haven't had regular ultrasounds or prenatal checkups.

Sure, it may feel like you've got two babies in there, especially if your baby is super-active, but as long as you're getting the proper prenatal care, you won't have any big surprises on D-day.

[#]105

What's wrong with kissing and snuggling with a cat or dog?

❑ a.   Pets may harbor infections that can be dangerous to your unborn baby.

❑ b.   Flea bites can be dangerous for your unborn baby.

❑ c.   Pets are more likely to bite you when you're pregnant.

❑ d.   Nothing—cuddle away. (Just don't touch any poop.)

Answer:
d.

Few infections can pass between people and animals. In fact, it's a lot more likely you'll catch a cold from snuggling with your significant other than from your pet.

Still, cats can carry a disease called toxoplasmosis that can be passed on to people via feline feces. For this reason, pregnant women should avoid changing cat litter or wear latex gloves and wash hands afterward.

Your doctor can do a simple blood test to check if you've already been exposed. If you have, no need to worry. If not, just take the following precautions:

- Change the box daily. The parasite does not become infectious until one to five days after it is shed in the cat's feces.
- Keep your cats inside. Indoor cats are less likely to become infected.
- Don't adopt or handle stray cats.
- Don't get a new cat while you're pregnant.
- Don't eat raw or undercooked meats.
- Don't feed raw or undercooked meat to your cats.

106

True or False:

Having a cat or dog as a pet while you're pregnant will increase your baby's chance of being allergic to animals.

Answer:

false.

Not only is it fine to have a cat or dog while you're pregnant, it may actually help your baby (as long as your pets don't bite, of course). Studies show that exposure to pets before and after birth can help reduce the chances of a baby later developing allergies and asthma. It's thought that pet exposure influences immunity development, in the womb and beyond.

And the more the merrier: A 2002 study funded by the National Institutes of Health found that children raised in homes with two or more dogs or cats were up to 77 percent less likely to have allergies than those raised without pets. Researchers think this protective effect may be the result of early exposure to bacteria carried by multiple pets. Exposing kids to such bacteria, it is thought, exercises their immune systems early in life, so they're better able to fight allergies later on.

Keep in mind that having a parent with allergies is still the biggest predictor of whether a child will be allergic too. Seven out of 10 kids with allergic parents will develop an allergy, compared to 1 out of 10 whose parents are allergy-free.

#107

Can I treat my dog for fleas?

❏ a.　No. Flea treatments can be toxic to your baby.

❏ b.　Yes, but have someone else apply a topical flea treatment.

❏ c.　Sure, just pick them off with a comb.

❏ d.　Yes, you can use electric currents to kill them.

Answer:

b.

It's fine to treat your pet for fleas, but it's a good idea to have someone else apply the medicine. Most topical flea solutions, flea baths, and flea collars contain pesticides that, in large doses, could be harmful to your unborn child. In the small amounts indicated for a single cat or dog, studies have shown no harmful effects, as long as you follow the manufacturer's directions. Flea-fighting pills, which circulate through your pet's bloodstream, are also safe.

If you're an animal groomer and work daily with pesticides, you might want to inquire about switching to a desk job, especially during your first trimester (when pesticide exposure is most harmful).

Or take a nontoxic route to fighting fleas. These methods may not be as effective, but they're better than nothing:

- Vacuum carpets, furniture, and floors regularly.
- Regularly wash all your pet's bedding, as well as rugs on which he frequently sleeps.
- Comb your pet daily with a metal flea comb.
- Boil six halved lemons in 1 quart of water. Steep overnight and then pour into a spray bottle. Spritz this natural flea fighter onto your pet, his bedding, and his favorite furniture.

108

True or False:

Cats are dangerous to newborn babies.

Answer:
false.

Those old wives' tales that cats will suck the life out of a baby or that cats will lay on top of a baby's face while he's sleeping are false. In fact, more babies and children have been killed by dogs, snakes, and even their own parents lying in bed next to them than by cats.

Such unfounded feline fears probably originated from these two truths:

1. Cats like to sniff people's breath (most likely, to relish the smells of recently eaten food).
2. Cats like to snuggle close to any warm object, whether a baby, a DVD player, or a sunny mantel.

There have been no substantiated cases of a cat killing a baby. Still, accidents do happen. In 1982, a British medical journal published a case of a 5-week-old baby found gasping for breath with a cat lying on her face. Her father performed mouth-to-mouth resuscitation, and she resumed breathing normally. Subsequently, she became sick and died of pneumonia seven months later. It was unclear whether the original incident caused her death, but it's enough of a tragedy to disconcert cat-owning parents. For this reason, it's never wise to allow your cat in the crib with your baby.

#109

Which of the following pets can be dangerous to my unborn baby?

- ❑ a. Dogs and cats.
- ❑ b. Turtles, snakes, and lizards.
- ❑ c. Rabbits, hamsters, and gerbils.
- ❑ d. Fish.

Answer:

b.

It might be time to find a new home for your pet turtle, snake, or lizard. These reptiles carry salmonella, a bacteria that can be dangerous for pregnant women and their babies. Though a salmonella infection doesn't usually affect the baby directly, the infection may cause severe diarrhea and vomiting in the mother, and that could cause a miscarriage. There is also a chance that the infection could cross the placenta, which may cause serious complications.

Salmonella is equally dangerous for children under 5 years, so hold off on reclaiming or replacing your reptiles until it's safe for your toddler.

Can't bear to part with your pet? Then take these precautions:

- Always wash hands thoroughly with soap and water after handling reptiles.
- Don't allow reptilian pets in the kitchen or near where you prepare food.
- Don't use the kitchen sink to clean your reptile's cage. If you use the bathtub, make sure to disinfect it afterward using a bleach solution.
- Don't allow young children to pet or hold reptiles.

#110

How can using a lubricant during prebirth sex affect my baby?

❑ a.   It can't.
❑ b.   It may contain chemicals harmful to your baby.
❑ c.   It may make you more likely to contract a sexually transmitted infection.
❑ d.   It may make your orgasms more intense, which can hurt your baby.

Answer:

a.

Lube away. Your cervix is tightly closed during pregnancy, which keeps any foreign materials (lube included) from reaching the uterus.

But choose wisely. During pregnancy, it's best to go with water-based lubricants, since they're less likely to irritate your vagina. And stay away from desensitizing and warming lubes, which often contain menthol or capsaicin (the spicy component of chili peppers). Since your skin is more sensitive during pregnancy, such formulas may irritate your vaginal area.

In fact, you may not need any lubricant at all, since vaginal discharge increases during pregnancy. Keep the bottle handy, though. After your baby is born, plummeting hormone levels may leave you uncomfortably dry south of the border.

111

Which of the following condoms are recommended for use during pregnancy?

❏ a.   Regular condoms.
❏ b.   Warming-sensation condoms.
❏ c.   Condoms with spermicide.
❏ d.   All of the above.

Answer:

a.

Condoms (both latex and latex-free) are safe to use during pregnancy. Just keep in mind that your skin—everywhere—is extra sensitive these days, so you may want to pass on the bells and whistles. Flavored condoms or those with warming sensations or spermicide, even if they used to work wonders for you, may now cause irritation.

Condom use is especially important if your partner has a sexually transmitted disease or infection, some of which can be transmitted to the baby before, during, or after birth. Diseases such as syphilis can cross the placenta and affect fetal development; gonorrhea, hepatitis B, and genital herpes can be transmitted to the baby during delivery and prove devastating to a newborn; and HIV can be transmitted through the placenta or during the birthing process. Avoid sex with a partner experiencing an active herpes outbreak, since that is when the virus is most contagious and condoms may not prevent its spread.

112

What can happen if my partner ejaculates inside me?

❏ a.   Nothing.
❏ b.   The hormones in sperm could affect your baby's sexual development.
❏ c.   The sperm could cause a miscarriage.
❏ d.   The hormones in sperm could jump-start labor.

Answer:

d.

Your cervix is tightly closed during pregnancy, which keeps foreign substances from entering your uterus and commingling with your baby. Your baby is also enclosed in a sac where the only things getting in do so through the umbilical cord. Suffice it to say, any sperm coming from your partner's penis won't even get into the uterus.

Still, semen contains hormones called prostaglandins—the same hormones doctors use to induce labor. Theoretically, exposure to semen late in pregnancy can trigger contractions; however, most doctors say the amount of prostaglandins contained in sperm can induce labor only when a woman is full term or overdue.

In addition, a study by scientists at the University of Adelaide in Australia found that regular exposure to a partner's sperm decreased the incidence of preeclampsia, a dangerous condition for both mother and baby. The reasons are not completely clear.

#113

Why do I sometimes cramp up after having sex during pregnancy?

❑ a.   Because the baby is overstimulated.
❑ b.   Because orgasms cause the uterus to contract.
❑ c.   Because sex exercises your abdominal muscles.
❑ d.   Because you may be going into labor.

Answer:

b.

The uterus naturally contracts when you have an orgasm.
These contractions happen even when you're not pregnant, but
it's just more noticeable when your uterus is bigger. As long as
you're having a normal pregnancy and haven't been advised
by your doctor to avoid sex or orgasms, these contractions are
harmless. They may make your belly look a little lopsided,
but they won't bother your baby. You may also notice slightly
painful cramping after sex, but that is also normal.

In most cases, the cramps will subside within 15 minutes
to an hour. Lying on your left side may help. Call your doctor if
the cramping or hardened feeling persists, if you start noticing
regular contractions, or if you have any unusual vaginal discharge or bleeding.

114

What happens if I use a vibrator during pregnancy?

❑ a.   The vibrations can rattle the baby.
❑ b.   The plastic can be toxic to the baby.
❑ c.   The orgasms are more intense, which can cause preterm labor.
❑ d.   Nothing.

Answer:
d.

The vibrations won't bother your baby at all. So, as long as
your doctor hasn't put you on pelvic rest (which means nothing
goes in the vagina) or told you to avoid orgasms, it's safe to use
a vibrator. Plus, the extra blood circulating in your vaginal
area during pregnancy may make your orgasms more intense
than ever.

Of course, you should always make sure that your sex toys
are clean and phthalate-free before using them. And be careful
not to insert any toy too forcefully or deeply, since plastic
doesn't bend as flesh does.

There are some conditions in which penetration and the
contractions created by orgasm may not be good for you. These
include

- placenta previa (when the placenta covers the cervix)
- previous early labor
- your water has broken
- you have a shortened cervix, or your cervix has shortened
  or dilated

115

True or False:

It's possible for the penis to hit the baby during deep penetration.

Answer:

false.

Even if your partner is extremely well endowed, his penis won't touch the baby during sex because your tightly closed cervix stands in its way. That said, he may bump up against your cervix, particularly during deep thrusts. The sensation may be painful, but it's not harmful. Try switching to a position in which you can control the depth of penetration (girl-on-top works well).

Don't panic if you notice a little spotting after sex. It's probably coming from your cervix, which can become irritated due to amped-up circulation and increased blood flow to the area. It's fairly common but nevertheless may be worth mentioning to your doctor, just to rule out any problems with your placenta (which can also cause bleeding).

As silly as it may sound, it's common for men to worry that their penises are getting too close to their offspring. And though such fears may lead to a temporary bout of abstinence, most women can safely have sex right up until the day they go into labor.

[#]116

Does my baby feel anything in utero when I have sex?

❏ a.   Yes, the baby may be squeezed during
          orgasm.
❏ b.   Yes, the baby may lose oxygen during sex.
❏ c.   Yes, the baby may be rocked to sleep by the
          movement.
❏ d.   No, the baby doesn't feel anything.

Answer:

C.

It's impossible to say for sure what a baby feels while his mother is engaging in sex because nobody's ever done studies to find out. Yet there's a good chance he feels something—but not much. All the movements you make are buffered by a bubble of amniotic fluid, so even if things get really raucous, your baby won't feel much of the action. The steady rhythm of your movements may even rock him to sleep, which is why many pregnant women say they feel fewer movements from their babies after sex.

Some experts also believe sex may give unborn babies a postcoital dose of the feel-good hormone oxytocin, which is released after orgasm. See that? It feels good for everyone.

#117

What effect can pregnancy have on my sex drive?

❑ a.   It increases it.
❑ b.   It decreases it.
❑ c.   It erases it.
❑ d.   All of the above.

Answer:

d.

Pregnancy affects women's sex drives differently. For most, the drive decreases in the first trimester, increases in the second, and then decreases again in the third. If yours is nowhere to be found, don't worry. It'll come back. (Sure, there may be a screaming baby down the hall making private time a bit more challenging, but you'll find a way.) For now, don't be too hard on yourself. Let's not forget you're growing a human being. There's a lot going on in your body—hormonal roller coaster notwithstanding—that can make having sex the last thing on your mind. And though some women can't get enough sex during pregnancy, others would rather watch the nursery paint dry than have their partners touch them.

Your hormones will return to their prepregnancy state about two or three months after your baby is born. (If you're breastfeeding, decreased estrogen levels put the kibosh on your libido, so your drive will return once your baby is weaned.) The fatigue of caring for a newborn might be another obstacle to the return of your sex life, but once parenthood becomes easier, you'll figure out how to work it all in. Two words: naptime quickies.

#118

Is it safe to receive oral sex while pregnant?

❑ a.   No, the mouth is full of germs, which can be transmitted to your baby via oral sex.

❑ b.   No, oral sex can cause intense orgasms that can cause early labor.

❑ c.   Yes, as long as your partner doesn't have an STD.

❑ d.   Yes, as long as your partner didn't just eat something spicy.

Answer:

C.

The mouth can be a dirty place, but unless your partner has a sexually transmitted infection such as gonorrhea, chlamydia, or syphilis (all of which can live in the mouth), receiving oral sex will not make you or your baby sick.

You should take a couple precautions, though:

Don't engage in oral sex if your partner has a cold sore. Cold sores are caused by the herpes virus, which can be spread to the genitals during oral sex. A herpes infection can be devastating to a baby, especially when contracted in the second and third trimesters, before your body has a chance to develop antibodies against the virus.

Make sure that your partner does not blow air into your vagina. It is possible (though extremely rare) for a burst of air to block a blood vessel and cause an embolism, which could be life-threatening to you and your baby. This could happen whether or not you're pregnant, but it's more of a risk during pregnancy because of increased blood flow to the vaginal area.

119

True or False:

Childbirth will change my vagina.

Answer:

true.

Your vagina must stretch to squeeze out that little human
being. It will shrink back after your baby is born but will
remain a little bit larger, especially if you delivered a big baby.
Most partners say they can't tell the difference, and it won't
feel any different to you. Doing daily Kegel exercises may help
you regain your prebaby tone. (For tips on performing Kegels,
see page 28.)

Don't expect to have sex right away: You should wait
six weeks to allow your cervix to close, postpartum bleeding
to stop, and any tears or stitches to heal. The vaginal tissue
may be tender and dry for up to several months after delivery,
so sex may hurt the first few times. C-section moms aren't
immune from sexual discomfort; studies show that they are
just as likely to suffer from painful sex after childbirth as
women who deliver vaginally.

For a minority of women, a feeling of "looseness" may
linger, especially after giving birth to a large baby or after
several vaginal births. This can be alleviated with daily Kegel
exercises or, in severe cases, vaginal surgery.

#120

Legally speaking, when must I tell a prospective employer that I'm pregnant?

- ❏ a.   During the initial interview.
- ❏ b.   During the final interview.
- ❏ c.   When you get the job offer.
- ❏ d.   Never.

Answer:

d.

Legally, you're not obligated to tell prospective employers you're pregnant, because your pregnancy has nothing to do with whether you're the right candidate for the job. That said, if you wait until after you're hired to disclose the big news, your boss may feel misled—and that's not a good way to start a professional relationship.

Interview for the job as usual, and when you enter the negotiation stage of the hiring process, discuss your pregnancy. Be honest about your expectations and future plans: Do you plan to send your child to daycare? Have you always planned on being a working mom?

It's illegal for a company to discriminate because of pregnancy. So if you're not hired because of your baby bump, or if a company rescinds its offer after you tell them you're expecting, you may have a lawsuit on your hands (though it might be difficult to prove).

#121

Can I defer jury duty because of my pregnancy?

❑ a.   Yes, pregnant women don't have to serve on juries.

❑ b.   Yes, but only if you have a doctor's note.

❑ c.   No, but you'll probably be dismissed since lawyers avoid assigning pregnant women to juries.

❑ d.   No, the court will not accept your pregnancy as an excuse.

Answer:
b.

Being pregnant is not a medical condition, so pregnancy itself can't excuse you from serving. However, if your doctor gives a medical reason explaining that you can't serve jury duty—you're on bed rest from an incompetent cervix, for instance—then you can be excused. Your doctor may also write a note if you're close to your due date and likely to go into labor in the courtroom.

Keep in mind that most states allow prospective jurors to postpone jury duty as long as they agree to serve at a later date; read the information on your summons for instructions. You may even be able to request a postponement online.

122

True or False:

An employer must allow you to take a leave of absence if you have severe morning sickness.

Answer:

true.

According to the U.S. Family and Medical Leave Act (FMLA), a woman is allowed to take up to 12 weeks of intermittent leave during pregnancy for a medical condition that makes her unable to do her job. Severe morning sickness qualifies, and a doctor's note is required.

The FMLA doesn't cover companies with fewer than 50 employees, and it guarantees only unpaid leaves. Whether you'll be paid for your time off is up to the state and your employer. Currently, California, Washington, and New Jersey are the only states to offer paid leave programs.

Talk to your human resources department or contact your state's Department of Labor to find out what you're entitled to.

#123

True or False:

Jobs that require long periods of standing, such as waiting tables, can be unhealthy for pregnant women after the third trimester.

Answer:

true.

According to a review of 29 studies involving more than 160,000 pregnant women, physically demanding work increased the chance of a woman delivering early (before 37 weeks) by 22 percent and increased her chance of developing hypertension or preeclampsia by 60 percent. Prolonged standing increased the risk of preterm birth by 26 percent.

Consequently, the American Medical Association recommends that women whose jobs have them on their feet for four or more hours a day should stop working or switch to less-demanding jobs by the 24th week of pregnancy, especially if they have a history of miscarriage or preterm births.

Granted, that's unrealistic for many women. But try asking your boss to be reassigned to different duties (greeting clients, for example). By law, employers can't fire women because they're pregnant; however, they don't have to pay those who take a leave of absence.

Can't afford to take time off? Rest between orders and take breaks whenever possible. And remember that the vast majority of women who work in the service industry have normal pregnancies and healthy babies.

124

Which of the following professions are dangerous for pregnant women?

- ❏ a.   Artist, agricultural worker, and dry cleaner.
- ❏ b.   X-ray attendant and lab worker.
- ❏ c.   Health care worker.
- ❏ d.   All of the above.

Answer:

d.

Though many women continue working as usual while pregnant, the following occupational hazards are worth noting.

Chemicals: Paint fumes, pesticides, carbon monoxide, oil paint, cigarette smoke, and other chemicals can harm a developing fetus. **Recommendation:** Wear an oxygen mask while working. Avoid exposure, especially during the first trimester.

Radiation: Evidence suggests that X-ray exposure may affect a developing fetus. **Recommendation:** Avoid contact with X-rays and nuclear radiation, especially during the first trimester.

Germs: Being around a person sick with a contagious infection is risky. **Recommendation:** Wash your hands frequently. Don't rub your eyes, nose, and mouth. Don't go to work if there's an outbreak. If you work in a medical or laboratory facility, wear gloves and a mask.

Physical demands: Physically strenuous work, especially in the third trimester, can increase your risk for preterm delivery, hypertension, and preeclampsia. **Recommendation:** Starting around the 24th week of pregnancy, stop working or find less demanding work. Take frequent breaks and rest.

#125

True or False:

Men can get morning sickness, too.

Answer:

true.

Though they're not the ones carrying and delivering the baby, up to 65 percent of men may experience symptoms like those of their expecting partners. Usually beginning around the third month of pregnancy, the symptoms include mood swings, cravings, fatigue, nausea, insomnia, weight gain, stomach cramps, and even a bloated belly.

This phenomenon is called couvade syndrome, and theories abound to explain it. Some experts believe it develops when a man, programmed to protect his family, realizes he can't do anything to alleviate his partner's pain. Since he can't "fix" the problem, he takes on some of it himself. Other scientists theorize that experiencing pregnancy symptoms is a man's instinctive display of commitment to his partner.

Recent studies suggest that men experience significant hormonal changes during their partners' pregnancies—specifically, higher levels of prolactin, a hormone associated with milk production in women and possibly maternal and paternal behavior. Men have also been found to have higher levels of estradiol, a form of estrogen, and decreased levels of testosterone. These changes may help men bond with their children, making them more likely to stick around for child rearing.

#126

Which of the following is true?

❑ a.   Pregnancy makes you more forgetful.
❑ b.   Pregnancy makes you dumber.
❑ c.   Pregnancy makes you smarter.
❑ d.   None of the above.

Answer:

C.

"Momnesia," also called "pregnant brain," is a myth. At least that's according to a 2008 Australian study that tracked 1,241 women before and after giving birth. Researchers gave the women a series of cognitive tests, first in 1999 and again in 2004 and 2008. They found no difference in brainpower during or after pregnancy.

In fact, pregnancy may even make you smarter. Studies of animals have found that mothers are braver, have better spatial awareness, and are up to five times faster at catching prey than their childless counterparts.

So what causes the absentmindedness experienced by many moms-to-be? Probably sleep deprivation. Getting a good night's sleep isn't easy during pregnancy, thanks to fluctuating hormones and a growing belly. It's also possible that your thoughts are too focused on your baby to remember little things like, say, where you parked your car.

#127

True or False:

A gush of fluid from the vagina is a surefire sign that labor is about to begin.

Answer:
false.

A soaked pair of skivvies could mean your water has broken . . .
or that you just wet your pants. How to tell the difference?
Check for these clues:

- **Duration:** If the leaking continues over a period of hours,
  it's probably amniotic fluid. Urine will stop once the
  bladder has been emptied.
- **Color and smell:** Amniotic fluid is usually clear and
  odorless (though it might have a slight salty smell).
- **Intensity:** If the fluid soaks through your clothes and
  continues to do so even after you've changed, it's amniotic
  fluid. Here's a good test: Change your underwear and then
  lie down for 30 minutes. If when you get up you feel a
  gush of liquid, most likely your sac has ruptured.
- **Consistency:** If you suspect your water has broken while
  you're urinating (a common occurrence), check the appearance and consistency of the liquid in the toilet bowl. Amniotic
  fluid may look oily and contain white specks.

Always call your doctor if you suspect your water has
broken.

#128

How can a mirror in the delivery room help during labor?

❑ a.   Seeing the baby's head crown can motivate you to keep pushing.

❑ b.   Seeing what the doctors are doing can make you feel at ease.

❑ c.   Seeing yourself in the throes of labor is comforting.

❑ d.   Seeing a different view of the action can distract you from the pain.

Answer:

a.

For some women, watching their babies make their entrances
into the world is something they wouldn't want to miss; for
others, it's a gory detail they'd rather not see. But witnessing
your baby's head peeking through the vaginal walls may be
worth the gore. Besides being an incredible sight to behold, this
first glimpse can motivate you to keep pushing, especially after
a long and exhausting labor.

If the idea still doesn't appeal to you, your doctor or
midwife can direct your hand to your vagina so that you can
touch the baby's head as it crowns. Or, you can receive play-
by-play reports. Just tell your doctor what you want—or don't
want—to see.

#129

What can I do to avoid pooping on the delivery room table?

❑ a.   Not much. Pooping is the norm, not the exception.

❑ b.   Ask your doctor to use an anal plug during delivery.

❑ c.   Take a laxative daily during your last three weeks of pregnancy to keep your bowels clean.

❑ d.   It's a myth that you'll poop during labor.

Answer:

a.

The pushing you do to deliver your baby is the same kind of pushing you do when going to the bathroom. In fact, most doctors consider it a good thing when women poop during labor, because it means they're pushing correctly. (You may pass gas, too.)

If you're really embarrassed about it, try increasing your fiber intake and drinking more water to reduce the likelihood that you'll push out more than just your baby. Taking a mild stool softener (found in some prenatal vitamins) throughout your pregnancy, especially during the last trimester, can also help.

You can also take an enema when labor starts. In the good old days, this practice was standard so that women could avoid the not-so-dainty act of defecating in front of their doctors. If you have time during the early phases of contractions, go for it. You can also request it when you check into the hospital, though many hospitals refuse because it could lead to dehydration, which may make labor more difficult.

In any event, whatever mess you make is nothing the doctors and nurses haven't seen before, and it will be cleaned up before you even know what's happened.

130

Which of the following may induce labor?

- ❑ a. Hanging upside down.
- ❑ b. Massaging your nipples.
- ❑ c. Listening to opera music.
- ❑ d. Watching videos of labor.

Answer:

b.

You can't do much to jump start labor (besides medical induction at a hospital). Your body will begin the process when it's time. But if your body is ready but your baby hasn't gotten the message, try the following:

Nipple stimulation: Massaging the nipples is believed to induce labor, though doctors say you'd have to do a few hours of daily nipple play to bring on the action.

Unprotected sex: Semen contains the same hormones given when doctors induce labor. However, don't have sex if your water has already broken, because it puts your baby at risk for infection.

Walking: If you're having contractions but not yet in full-blown labor, walking may help get the show on the road.

Acupuncture/acupressure: Two pressure points are believed to cause contractions in the uterus: one located on your inner calf, about two inches above your ankle, and the other in the webbed space between your thumb and forefinger. To stimulate these points, pinch or rub in a circular motion for 30 to 60 seconds. Wait several minutes and repeat.

Lightning Round Questions:

131. How early was the world's most premature baby?

    a. 74 days early   *c.* 128 days early

    b. 110 days early   *d.* 156 days early

132. When does a baby's heart start beating?

    a. The moment of conception   *c.* The fifth week of pregnancy

    b. The first week of pregnancy   *d.* The 12th week of pregnancy

133. How much weight does the average man gain during his partner's pregnancy?

    a. 5 pounds   *c.* 20 pounds

    b. 14 pounds   *d.* 30 pounds

134. At what age do scientists believe babies develop preferences for the right or left hand?

    a. The 12th week of pregnancy   *c.* The 34th week of pregnancy

    b. The 25th week of pregnancy   *d.* As a toddler

135. What percentage of women get stretch marks?

    a. 10 percent   *c.* 75 percent

    b. 25 percent   *d.* 90 percent

136. What percentage of babies are born on their due dates?

    a. 1 percent   *c.* 8 percent

    b. 5 percent   *d.* 10 percent

137. How large at birth was the world's smallest surviving baby?

    a. 2.5 ounces   *c.* 9.5 ounces

    b. 8.6 ounces   *d.* 12.1 ounces

138. True or False: First-time mothers are more likely to deliver past their due dates.

139. What percentage of U.S. babies are born to unmarried women?

    a. 20 percent   *c.* 60 percent

    b. 40 percent   *d.* 75 percent

140. What percentage of women work through their pregnancies?

    a. 25 percent   *c.* 67 percent

    b. 42 percent   *d.* 82 percent

141. True or False: Boy babies outnumber girl babies.

142. Which are the most popular months for babies to be born in the United States?

    a. July through September   *c.* December through February

    b. March through May   *d.* October through December

143. Which is the most popular day for babies to be born in the United States?

    a. Monday   *c.* Thursday

    b. Tuesday   *d.* Sunday

144. What is the average age of first-time mothers in the United States?

    a. 21   *c.* 27

    b. 25   *d.* 29

145. What percentage of pregnancies in the U.S. are unplanned?

    a. 22 percent   *c.* 62 percent

    b. 48 percent   *d.* 80 percent

146. What percentage of births in the U.S. are delivered by C-section?

    a. 10 percent   *c.* 32 percent

    b. 17 percent   *d.* 45 percent

147. Which of the following senses can be altered by pregnancy?

    a. taste   *c.* sight

    b. smell   *d.* all of the above

148. How much weight does the average woman gain during pregnancy?

    a. 15 pounds   *c.* 30 pounds

    b. 20 pounds   *d.* 40 pounds

149. What is the highest number of babies born to one woman?

a. 16   *c.* 69

b. 34   *d.* 78

150. Despite the danger that cigarette smoke poses to unborn babies, what percentage of U.S. mothers smoke during their pregnancies?

a. 45 percent   *c.* 15 percent

b. 25 percent   *d.* 10 percent

Answers:

146. *c.*	147. *d.*	148. *c.*	149. *c.*	150. *d.*
141. *true.*	142. *a.*	143. *b.*	144. *b.*	145. *b.*
136. *b.*	137. *b.*	138. *true*	139. *b.*	140. *c.*
131. *c.*	132. *c.*	133. *b.*	134. *b.*	135. *d.*

Index